Plant Based Cookbook

A Complete Meal Prep Guide with Quick and Easy Recipes for Healthy Eating and to Reset and Energize Your Body and Mind

Sophia Scott

Legal & Disclaimer

The information contained in this book and its contents is not designed to replace or take the place of any form of medical or professional advice; and is not meant to replace the need for independent medical, financial, legal or other professional advice or services, as may be required. The content and information in this book has been provided for educational and entertainment purposes only.

The content and information contained in this book has been compiled from sources deemed reliable, and it is accurate to the best of the Author's knowledge, information and belief. However, the Author cannot guarantee its accuracy and validity and cannot be held liable for any errors and/or omissions. Further, changes are periodically made to this book as and when needed. Where appropriate and/or necessary, you must consult a professional (including but not limited to your doctor, attorney, financial advisor or such other professional advisor) before using any of the suggested remedies, techniques, or information in this book.

Table of Contents

INTRODUCTION

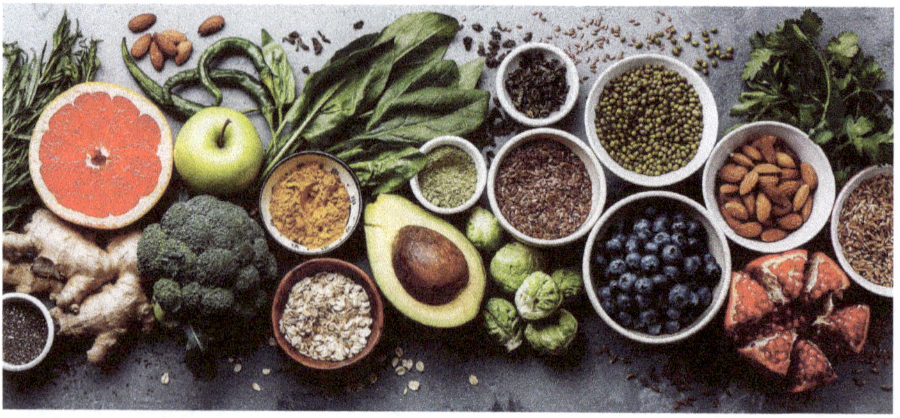

What is Whole-Food, Plant-Based?

The plant-based diet emphasizes on eating both fresh and whole ingredients. Basically, you are going to want to avoid food that has been highly processed. By eating minimally processed foods and increasing the plants in your diet, it will be effective in helping you to lose weight, improve your health, or both!

There is no true definition of the plant-based diet because it is so much more than a diet. Most diets set you up for failure. If you're anything like me, you must have tried a handful of them already. Many individuals follow strict rules like cutting sugar, cutting carbs, or completely eliminating food groups that they love. Unfortunately, it's hard to do it this way because it's hard to just drop your bad habits. On the other hand, a plant-based diet doesn't have strict rules like these. Instead, it has basic principles that anyone can follow on their own time and pace. The best part is that it is inclusive, so you can make this lifestyle a family event!

Often, a plant-based diet is confused with a vegan or vegetarian diet. While they are very similar, they are not exactly the same. The best way to describe it is that a plant-based diet is the umbrella term where veganism and vegetarianism fall under. A plant-based diet is extremely versatile to help fit the needs of a variety of people. Yes, there is an emphasis on whole foods that have been minimally processed, but technically, animal products are still allowed on this diet, though they should be limited!

Instead of focusing on the foods that you can't have, you'll be encouraged to learn how to enjoy new types of food such as nuts, seeds, legumes, whole grains, fruits, and vegetables. Later in the chapters of this book, you'll even be provided with a grocery list, meal plan, and the foods you should avoid and the foods you should enjoy. As I said, I'm setting you up for complete success here! When we do this together, we'll also be able to save our planet one healthy person at a time.

Unfortunately, a plant-based diet is often thought of as boring and bland. While for some people, avoiding animal ingredients is incredibly limiting, you'll soon find out that as you become more innovative with your cooking skills, you will learn to create new flavors. As you try out some of the recipes provided in the next chapters, you'll discover flavors you did not know were even possible.

In order to understand the diet, it's important that you first understand its definition. When I say whole food, it simply refers to foods that are in their natural state. This means that the foods included on this diet are minimally refined, unrefined, or whole and raw.

As for the word "plant-based", this just means the bulk or base of your meal is primarily coming from plants. However, when I say "plant-based foods", this means the food comes directly from plant sources. We will be going over in greater detail in the next section but all you need to know at this point is that plant-based foods do not contain any animal products like honey, eggs, milk or meat. If you are thinking: "Oh, that is the majority of my diet!"; don't worry, you are not alone! That's because you've been brought up on S.A.D, also known as the Standard American Diet, which is the diet of most Americans. While switching to a plant-based diet may take some extra work, it is absolutely worth it because you're doing it for your health and the health of the environment.

Of course, thinking about moving to this diet is going to be your first step. While it sounds like an excellent idea, often it is difficult to know where to start. The next few chapters will introduce you to the incredible benefits of the diet, who it is for, and some tips and tricks to help you get started.

What Are Plant Foods?

You will see me refer to "plant foods" many times throughout this book. When I say, "plant food," I simply mean food that isn't from an animal in any shape or form. Some of the foods include potatoes, fruits, vegetables, legumes, mushrooms and more.

Some types of foods that are often confused with plant-based foods are plant fragments and plant-based processed foods. These are refined foods including chips, oil, sugar, and all-purpose flour. While these foods technically come from plants and do not contain any animal products, they are not considered plant foods. Plant foods must be whole or minimally processed.

You might be scratching your head at this point; I will clarify with an example. An apple is considered a plant food. An apple pie is not a plant food, nor is it plant-based. That is because typically, pies are prepared with milk and eggs. Another example is frozen corn. Frozen corn is considered a plant food while high fructose corn syrup is not because the syrup contains a high amount of processed sugar. Get the picture?

What Does Plant-Based Mean?

If someone tells you that they follow a plant-based diet, this means that their diet consists mainly of plant foods. Unless you are told otherwise, you can assume that this individual avoids animal-based products like gelatin, butter, milk, eggs, and animal meat, or they eat them very minimally. These individuals will also avoid eating plant fragments and place their focus on whole plant foods instead.

There will be a learning curve if you're just starting this diet but that does not mean it is impossible. You'd even be surprised to learn which foods are plant-based and which are not. While you may need to give up some of your favorite treats, I assure you there are some delicious alternatives out there. One of my favorite aspects of a plant-based diet is that you won't have to count calories. In fact, your diet will be filled to the brim with so many nutrient-dense foods that you'll never go hungry again, provided you're following the diet the correct way.

Minimally Processed Plant-based Foods

I know a lot of new terms are being thrown at you right now. Although it is a lot to take in at first, keep holding on. You will soon be a plant-based expert! You must understand all of these terms before diving into the diet so that you are well prepared for success. Knowledge truly is a powerful concept when it comes to succeeding with anything in life.

While you may think you understand what minimally processed means, you may be surprised to find that certain foods are more processed than you thought. Some examples are granola bars, corn tortillas, and breakfast cereals. While they are technically accepted as plant-based, they are actually highly processed. Just check out their labels and you'll see.

Some foods that are more minimally processed include oatmeal, peanut butter, salsa, applesauce, hummus, and even guacamole. Condiments like vinegar, soy sauce, hot sauce, and mustard are also considered minimally processed.

Two food items that cause a bit of confusion are mushrooms and yeast. While they are not technically considered plants, they can be consumed on a plant-based diet.

Another food that is often questioned is bread. While bread is suitable for most plant-based eaters, you will need to read its nutrient label to make a better judgment. Some kinds of bread that are sold commercially could potentially contain stabilizers, fillers, eggs and dairy. Obviously, this would mean that the bread is no longer fully plant-based. Luckily, there are many different types of bread out there for you to try that are still within the guidelines of your diet.

Plant-Based Diet Reference

As the plant-based diet grows in popularity and is being introduced to a wider audience, some people have modified and created different versions of it to fit their needs. The following diets are the most common ones.

- **Veganism**

  Veganism is a diet that includes only seeds, nuts, grains, legumes, and vegetables. Often, you will hear vegan and plant-based being used interchangeably. Later, we will be going over why they are not necessarily the same thing. However, in a nutshell, veganism is a lifestyle choice where an individual chooses to have no animal sources in their life from clothing to food choices.

  There are two main categories of veganism at this point. First, you have fruitarianism; this is a diet that consists primarily of fruit. The second is raw veganism. A raw vegan will eat foods that are uncooked or dehydrated. Obviously, both of these are very restrictive for a beginner, which is not what a plant-based diet should be.

- **Vegetarianism**

  A vegetarian will eat foods such as seeds, nuts, fruits, legumes, and vegetables, much like a vegan. They are similar in that they both do not eat meat. The main difference between a vegetarian and a vegan is that vegetarians still include eggs and dairy in their diet. There are several types of vegetarianism including ovo-lacto; includes dairy and eggs, ovo; includes eggs but no dairy, and lacto; which includes dairy but no eggs. You also have semi-vegetarians who eat mostly a vegetarian diet but will have meat on special occasions.

Another version of the vegetarian diet is the macrobiotic diet. This diet consists of naturally processed foods, sea vegetables, beans, vegetables, and whole grains.

- **Pescetarianism**

  There is also the pescatarian who follows a semi-vegetarian diet but includes seafood, dairy, and eggs.

As you can see, there're many different alternatives. Although a plant-based diet is not an easy change if you've had the average American diet for the longest time, its flexibility makes it perfectly do-able. As I've stated earlier, you are being provided with all of the information you need in this book to help get you started! At the end of the day, the responsibility still rests on your shoulders to put in the work and tailor your diet according to your needs and desires.

Plant-Based Benefits for the Environment

In the next chapter, you will be learning all the incredible health benefits the plant-based diet can bring you, but it is so much bigger than that. When you switch your lifestyle to being plant-based, you are also helping to save the environment. At the end of the day, what better gift can you give your children and loved ones than a cleaner and more beautiful environment to prosper in? With so much destruction in the world today, why not do your part?

For those of us who love our planet, it is a very scary world out there! Animal and plant habitats alike are being destroyed by deforestation. On top of that, we're facing global warming. By switching to a plant-based diet, you will be cutting down your carbon footprint and helping to protect the earth for future generations to come. You would be amazed to learn how much the animal-based industry of agriculture adds to our poor earth's woes. In fact, the factory farms in the United States produce about 300 million tons of waste every year! On top of that, these farms are also polluting our air and making us sicker than ever before. If you care about the environment, there are several ways a plant-based diet can help.

Cut Your Carbon Footprint

As of right now, the United Nations Food and Agriculture Organization has estimated that the production of livestock is responsible for a whopping 14.5% of global greenhouse gas emissions. It is believed that just cattle alone, which are raised for beef and milk, are responsible for 65% of these emissions. The other sources of these emissions come from feed processing and production to keep these animals alive.

As mentioned earlier, these animals produce about 300 million tons of waste per year. This waste is responsible for 37% of the agricultural greenhouse gas emissions. It is believed that there is a management factory farm referred to as lagoons where there are cesspits filled to the brim with this animal waste. This waste produces large quantities of methane, which is responsible for warming the earth about 20 times faster than carbon dioxide.

By switching over to a plant-based diet, you are massively decreasing or even totally cutting out animal products from your diet. In other words, you are reducing your carbon footprint by not contributing to this industry. While it may not seem like much, if everyone plays his or her individual part, it can make a significant difference.

Start Conserving Water

For most diets, it isn't specified clearly what beverages are recommended. Well, on the plant-based diet, a beverage you should be cutting down on will be milk. According to the Water Footprint Network, they have estimated that it takes around 1000 gallons of water to produce 1 gallon of milk. Also, it takes up to 6 times more water to produce 1 pound of animal protein compared to 1 pound of grain protein. More water is also needed for animal produce versus plant produce. The Twente Water Centre from the University of Twente has calculated that beef uses approximately 20 times more water than grains or potatoes.

When you go on a plant-based diet, you'd be reducing consumption of animal-products and thus, help to reduce the amount of water being used. You see, water is a very precious resource. What would happen if our children have to live in a world with no fresh water? That is why we need to pave the road towards a healthier planet today, for the sake of our future generations. At this point, it is no longer just about you or me. We must do what is best for the future of the entire human race.

Cleaner Air

Clean air is incredibly important. This is a resource that we all need to survive. Humans need it; animals need it, planet earth needs it. The manure from livestock is producing a potent form of nitrogen, more commonly referred to as ammonia. This ammonia is killing off algae, fish, and even adds smog into our cities. Studies have also found that the air surrounding factory farms have above-average levels of carbon dioxide, endotoxins, and hydrogen sulfide, and all of these are terrible for our environment. Again, switching to a plant-based diet means that you'll be helping to alleviate all these toxins from our planet.

Love Animals, Don't Eat Them!

One of the major reasons people succeed in switching to veganism or vegetarianism is due to their deep love for animals. If you are like me and you can't stand the thought of eating a living being that has some form of intelligence and sentience, then cutting animal protein out of your diet should be pretty easy. That's not all. On top of saving the animals, you'll also be helping to save the habitats of these animals. Animal agriculture is a huge contributor to desertification and deforestation of our planet. Studies have shown that animal agriculture takes about one-third of the arable land in the world. By taking up and damaging so much natural land, we could eventually see the extinction of many animal species such as sloths, red pandas, and orangutans.

The Power of Plant-based

While the animal agriculture does make up the core of our environmental issues, there are other factors leading to global warming and greenhouse gas emissions too. Similarly, there're several other contributing factors to land degradation, deforestation, and extinction. While it all does seem rather bleak, make no mistake that you still have the power to make a difference.

Two of the biggest problems we face today are global warming and eating ourselves to more diseases and even our deaths. However, the real problem is that most people are unwilling to do anything about it.

What many people do not know is that we can fight against climate change, and it happens to start right on our plates. By making proper food choices, we are taking back control of our own survival, all while creating true sustainability for future generations to come.

While we may be unable to change the future of our world overnight, we cannot underestimate the power of everyday habits. By choosing one plant-based meal today, it increases the odds of you choosing a plant-based meal tomorrow and then another plant-based meal the day after. As you begin to eat healthier, you're contributing to the demand and supply for plant produce. This ensures that vital crop resources are being prioritized to feed human beings as opposed to livestock. It also lets farmers know that plant produce is in-demand and a lucrative alternative to animal products. The more people switch to a plant-based diet, the more available plant-based options will be made for us. As individuals come together, I believe we truly will be able to make a difference in this world.

Of course, these are long-term benefits. However, a plant-based diet can also benefit your personal life right now. In the next chapter, you'll be learning just how efficiently whole foods can change your life for the better. From weight loss to improving your health conditions, a plant-based diet can change your life in ways you never even expected.

CHAPTER 1: THE PLANT-BASED DIET

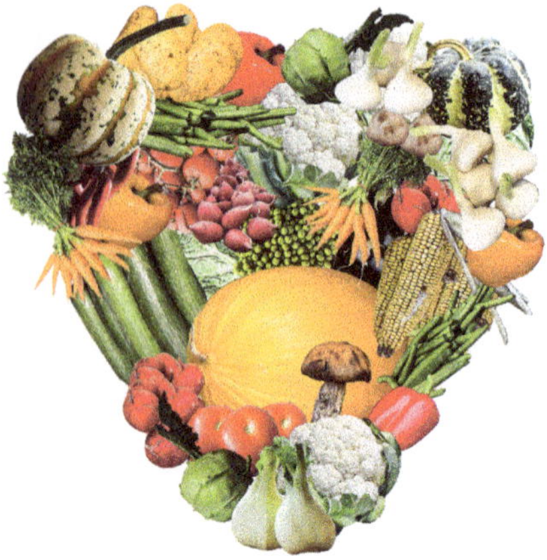

One of the main reasons that urge people to switch to a plant-based diet is the fact that it has so many wonderful and amazing health benefits. When you cut out all of the bad, processed food from your diet and replace it instead with whole, unrefined, and carefully-sourced plant products, you feel the benefits almost immediately. In fact, the healthy change is really what keeps most people on the diet. There is so much motivation to stay within the parameters of a plant-based diet when you are actually feeling better, healthier, and have more energy and stamina. Who would want to go back to eating unhealthily and feeling slow and sluggish after getting a taste of what your life on plant-based foods is like? And as a bonus, you can set your conscience at ease and know that you are taking the steps towards making a better, more protected planet. The plant-based diet is without a doubt one of the most environmental ways of eating you could choose.

There is no denying that we are in the midst of a crisis of chronic diseases like high cholesterol, diabetes, and high-blood pressure. Many people blame the almost universal shift to eating foods that are processed and animal-sourced like refined grains, sugar, salt, meat, oil, dairy, soda, and eggs. Most of the time, these foods are high in fat and low in nutritional value but we keep reaching for them all the same. However, there most certainly is hope. Plant-based diets are becoming much more mainstream and popular amongst people looking to improve their health and lengthen their lifespans. There are so many more products on the market geared towards helping people achieve a healthy, plant-based diet lifestyle than there used to be. Nowadays, you can easily find entire restaurants devoted to serving healthy plant-based meals and health food stores are a dime a dozen. It is easier than ever to switch to a plant-based diet. And that most certainly is good news for you.

We know for a fact that a plant-based diet is a healthier choice than eating lots of processed foods and animal products. Extensive research has been done on this topic. In one study, researchers used vegetarians who had lapsed from their diets as their main focus group. They found that people who used to subscribe to a vegetarian diet but fell out of it and began to eat meat at least once a week experienced an extremely raised risk of heart disease, stroke, diabetes, and weight gain. Studying them for 12 years after they transitioned away from a vegetarian diet, researchers found that life-expectancy was decreased as well. In studies where researchers put certain groups afflicted with diseases like heart disease, high cholesterol, or high blood pressure on an interventional plant-based diet, they found significant increases in satisfaction and health. These groups placed on plant-based diets reported that they were happier with their diet, had increased energy, better digestion, improved sleep, and overall better general and mental health. A plant-based diet has been proven to lower body weight, reduce sugar levels, and aids the body in controlling cholesterol levels. It also helps deal with your emotional and mental health. Many people who switch to a plant-based diet claim to experience a lessening of afflictions such as anxiety, fatigue, and depression. It gives many a greater sense of well-being and makes day-to-day functioning easier and more enjoyable.

Because switching to a plant-based diet increases your intake of potassium-rich foods, most people experience lower blood-pressure almost automatically. Whole grains, nuts, seeds, legumes, and fruits and vegetables all contain a great deal of potassium which directly targets blood pressure and lowers it while a lot of meats and animal products lack potassium and can actually pose the risk of raising cholesterol and blood pressure. These good plant foods also contain great amounts of vitamin B6, which helps lower blood pressure as well. With lower blood pressure comes decreased stress and anxiety. It's a win-win! And since blood pressure and cholesterol tend to be tandem, symbiotic issues, it is important to note that plants do not contain any cholesterol. Therefore, a plant-based diet is a kind of foolproof way to lower your cholesterol. High cholesterol and blood pressure are dangerous factors that lead to heart disease, the number one killer of adults in the United States. A plant-based diet thus lowers your risk of heart disease because it ensures that you are putting better, healthier foods into your body that will not make your blood pressure and cholesterol levels skyrocket like some of the other fatties, processed foods and animal products out there.

Followers of a plant-based diet also experience better blood sugar levels. The simplest way to combat high blood sugar is to consume more fiber as is slows the absorption of sugar into the bloodstream. Plant foods and whole grains are incredibly high in fiber while animal products have been proven to raise blood sugar to unhealthy and at times dangerous levels. More balanced blood sugar helps prevent type 2 diabetes and results in a much healthier life. Whole foods that are nutritious and low in fat also greatly decrease your risk of cancer. Some animal products such as cured meats are thought to be linked to the development of certain cancers. With a plant-based diet, your chances of having cancer are much lowered than someone who does not subscribe to a plant-based diet. It is for these many reasons that many doctors actually champion the plant-based diet and recommend it to patients who are overweight or afflicted with high cholesterol, high blood pressure, or other cardiovascular troubles. Plant-based diets have been shown time and time again to be economical and low-risk ways to make a significant change in one's health for the better. Switching to a plant-based diet may help lower the body mass index (BMI) in addition to blood pressure and cholesterol levels. Because of this, patients may need to take fewer medications to treat their illnesses, thus cutting out unnecessary expenses and the need to take many pills. All of these heart-healthy benefits also manifest themselves in the form of weight management and appetite control, all of which we will delve further into in the next chapter.

When you begin to feel immensely healthier due to all the benefits of a plant-based diet, your mental and emotional health will inevitably follow along. Many people notice improved sleeping patterns after making the switch. Not only do they sleep more regularly, the sleep deeper and better. Sleep is so important to our mental and physical health and unfortunately it is usually one of the first things we sacrifice in our daily lives. There are deadlines to be met, tasks to be completed, and things to do- it can all get overwhelming. When do we have time to sleep? And when we do, is it a good sleep? Switching to a plant-based diet can really help you get in control of your sleep and maximize the actual benefits of your pillow time. Eating plant-based makes the body a well-oiled machine and as such, it becomes more able to recharge itself efficiently. Therefore, you get the most out of your precious, valuable time for sleep. Better sleep can lead to a significant increase in the quality of one's mental health. A good night's sleep elevates mood and boosts energy so that you can be more productive and motivated during the day.

In addition to the many medical benefits of switching to a plant-based diet, there are also some truly powerful and indisputable cosmetic benefits as well. Many studies have shown that there is a significant and strong link between the consumption of dairy products like milk, butter, or cheese, and undesirable skin conditions like acne, eczema, and early signs of aging. Milk contains many similar properties to the hormone testosterone due to other hormones like progesterone making their way into the milk. It is thought that these hormones stimulate the oil glands of the skin, especially the face. An excess of sebum, or oil, is produced and thus acne occurs. This excess oil clogs your pores and can lead to other troublesome skin blemishes such as blackheads and whiteheads. This continuous cycle of clogged pores, blemishes, and acne takes a lot out of your skin and can cause scarring and stress. This can lead to signs of premature aging and skin loses its elasticity and vitality. Many people who switch to a plant-based diet notice an incredibly rapid improvement in the condition of their skin. People who have suffered from acne and started eating plant-based foods have noticed their skin clear significantly. This is in no way by chance. Cutting out or greatly reducing dairy can really help give your skin a new lease on life. If you are struggling with acne and have tried nearly everything under the sun such as harsh chemicals, expensive facials and skin treatments, or countless different brands claiming to heal your skin problems, something as simple as a plant-based diet may be the answer you've been searching for.

Followers of a plant-based diet have also raved about the excellent anti-aging benefits of the diet. Collagen, something our bodies naturally produce in abundance when we are young, is the key factor of what makes skin supple, resilient and firm. As we get older, collagen production slows and our skin suffers as a result, becoming prone to sagginess and thinness. While this is a natural and inevitable part of life, collagen loss does not have to be so drastic as we age. A plant-based diet has been proven to boost collagen in your body by providing all of the important nutrients and amino acids that make up collagen and how it is produced. In a sense, subscribing to a plant-based diet is kind of like taking a dip in the fountain of youth! Fruits and vegetables like kale, broccoli, asparagus, spinach, grapefruit, lemons, and oranges are chock-full of vitamin C, which is an extremely important component in producing the amino acids that make up collagen. The kind of lean protein found in nuts is important in keeping collagen around, adding to skin cell longevity and resilience. Red vegetables like tomatoes, beets, and red peppers all contain lycopene, which is a kind of antioxidant that protects skin from the sun while simultaneously increases collagen production. Foods rich in zinc such as certain seeds and whole grains also promote collagen because the mineral repairs damaged cells and reduces inflammation. So many of the plant-based staples contain incredible amounts of all these collagen-boosting nutrients that you do not even have to go out of your way to seek them out. It is all right there in front of you! Looking and feeling younger has never been so easy. It really does start with the internal to make the external radiant and glowing, outer beauty starts from within.

In short, there are no two ways about it - switching to a plant-based diet is good for your heart, your health, your mind, and even your physical appearance! The facts of the matter are undeniable. Plant foods contain so many of the incredibly good nutrients that our bodies need to function properly. Making these foods a priority and centering your meals around them rather than just eating vegetables as an occasional side dish or a piece of fruit every now and then makes a huge difference in your health. By eating a diet heavy on meat, dairy, and other animal products and processed foods, it is easy to miss out on the wonderfully beneficial vitamins, minerals, antioxidants, and other nutrients that are in fruits, vegetables, legumes, tubers, grains, nuts, and seeds. Switching to a plant-based diet allows you to obtain all of these healthful ingredients that will without a doubt lead you to a better, more fulfilling life.

WHAT TO EAT

Eating restrictions are pretty easy to understand in this diet. There is a wide range of whole plant-based products allowed in the diet. In this way, you will be receiving a great variety to try new dishes.

What to eat in a plant-based diet:

- Fruits: All kinds of whole fruits are allowed in this diet. You just have to have fruits in their organic form. Don't use fruit juices or dried fruits and other refined options.
- Vegetables with no starch: All vegetables are allowed in the diet such as leafy greens, zucchini, broccoli, tomatoes, eggplant, and others.
- Vegetables with starch: Vegetables with starch content are also accepted in this diet. So, you can utilize potatoes, legumes, sweet potatoes, beans, corn, peas, plantains, squash, and others.
- Whole grains: All whole grains with 100% purity are allowed in this diet. You can utilize brown rice, whole wheat, oats, and other whole grain choices in your plant-based diet.
- Beverages: In the category of beverages, you can only use plant-based milk without any sweetness. Also, water, tea, coffee, and green tea are allowed options in this diet.
- Spices: All kinds of spices are accepted in the plant-based diet.

- Sources of omega-3: All safe sources of omega-3 are promoted during the plant-based diet. So, you are motivated to include flax seeds, chia seeds, and other resources in your meals.

WHAT TO AVOID

- Meat: All kinds of meat products such as fish, seafood, poultry, red meat, and even processed meat products are not allowed in a plant-based diet.
- Eggs: You can't eat eggs, as it contains high cholesterol content.
- Dairy: All forms of dairy products are not accepted in this diet. You have to avoid milk, cream, cheese, buttermilk, and half-and-half.
- Vegan replacements: Vegan replacements of meats and cheese are also not allowed. Such replacements contain high oil content, which is not acceptable in the plant-based diet.
- Added fat: You have to say no to all kinds of added fats such as coconut oil, butter, margarine, and all other liquid oils.
- Refined flours: Any flour that is not 100% in terms of whole wheat is not accepted. You can't use refined flours in your diet.

- Added sugar: Any food item with added flavoring or sugar is not allowed. Along with that, you have to say no to energy bars, candy bars, cakes, cookies, and all other junk food options.
- Beverages: In the category of beverages, you can't have soda or even fruit juices. Even the fruit juices with 100% purity are not allowed. At the same time, you are recommended to stay away from energy drinks, sports drinks, tea drinks, blended coffee, and other harmful beverages that contain flavorings or high-sugar content.

Shopping List

Fresh vegetables and fruits: Look for all varieties of fresh vegetables and fruits you can find. Give priority to leafy greens.

Legumes and beans: Dried lentils and beans have multiple varieties available in the market. You can use them all. Just make sure you rinse them before using.

Seeds and nuts: Nuts take the place of liquid oils in your meals. However, you can avoid nuts if you want to lose weight or have a heart condition. Choose seeds of chia and flax to intake high omega-3 content. Similarly, you can purchase other seeds such as sesame, sunflower, and pumpkin.

Whole grain bread and tortillas: For enchiladas, tacos, burritos, burgers, and other cooking options, you will require whole grain versions of bread and tortillas. Make sure you find 100% pure whole grain buns, tortillas, and bread in the market.

Whole grains: The choices of whole grains include quinoa, brown rice, cornmeal, oatmeal, and others. But you need to focus on the wholegrain quality of the choices you pick.

Pasta and noodles of brown rice: Pasta and noodles of brown rice will help you make some great pasta recipes in different varieties.

Cereals for breakfast: When buying cereals, you have to avoid sweetened ones and the ones that contain added oils. Pick whole grain cereals such as rolled oats, steel cut options of oatmeal, bran flakes, and/or grape nuts.

Plant-based milk: Nondairy substitutes are required from time to time to gain the smoothness in dishes.

You can purchase almond milk, rice milk, soy milk, cashew milk, and other plant-based milk. However, ensure that no milk option contains added flavors or sugars. Also, stay away from products that contain added oils in their milk.

Pasta and tomato sauce and salsa: Salsa and sauce are a great option when you are cooking pasta. When buying these products, you have to ensure the absence of any animal food content, added oils, and/or sugar content.

Food processor or blender: A food processor or a blender would be a helpful option when you are cooking vegetable soups or making homemade salsa. So, purchase a high-quality machine to process food items.

With that, you are now ready to begin your plant-based diet. All you need now is some great recipes, to begin with. So, let's give you a list of breakfast, soups, salads, and main meal recipes.

TIPS AND TRICKS FOR REAL LIFE

Switching over to a new diet can be very intimidating, especially if you are just starting out. If you're anything like me, I know you've either been eating the same unhealthy way all your life, or you have been bouncing from diet to diet searching for answers. I hope I've provided enough value to you so far such that you're convinced that the plant-based diet is truly beneficial for you and your loved ones! However, I love to provide you with even more value. Thus, to ensure you really feel comfortable moving forward, I've included some of my favorite tips to help you get started and stay motivated!

Believe in Yourself

Although there are many misconceptions about the plant-based diet, do not let them distract you. Believe in your food choices and just keep going, slowly you'll find that the plant-based lifestyle will become more and more abundant in your life. Even on your first trip to the grocery store on a plant-based diet, you'll begin to notice all the vegan products available.

I am a true believer that 80% of any success story is having the right mindset. A big part of this mindset is having self-belief and to fully trust the process! Self-belief will also guide you in making decisions that are aligned with your goals. To help you get into this winning mindset, I just want to remind you that you're already way ahead of the pack because you have this book of knowledge. That's an incredible advantage for you to take back control of your life.

Take Small Bites

I mean this literally and figuratively. Nobody is expecting you to change your diet cold turkey. I don't want you to wake up tomorrow morning and tell yourself, "no more animal products forever!" Unfortunately, this will only cause you to panic and binge. Instead, I suggest you give up one item at a time. Perhaps to begin, try eating a plant-based meal once or twice a week. As you become more comfortable with this new way of eating, you can then take the next step of replacing more food items in your diet.

At the beginning, when you're trying to reduce the consumption of meat, it's very normal to fall back into your old eating habits. If that happens, you can help yourself by reducing the amount of meat you are eating in a week instead of in a day. The same goes for dairy and egg products. When you take smaller steps, it does not raise your chance of following through; it also boosts your confidence as you make these small wins along the way. As time goes on, you'd be surprised to learn that everything feels much easier.

Say Goodbye to Labels

For some reason, we feel the need to label everything and everyone. You'll get many people trying to put you in a box by calling you a vegan or vegetarian and segregating you from the others based on your diet choice. You might feel left out sometimes. However, do not mind them. Let people label you however way they want. As long as you stay strong and do not let it deter you from staying on your plant-based diet, you're on your way to a healthier and happier life. In the end, trying is better than not attempting at all!

As you begin to make healthier food choices, it's normal to slip up. I don't want you to go into this lifestyle expecting to be perfect. Focus on progress instead of perfection. Don't label yourself as well because that's putting too much pressure on you. If you become too strict on yourself, your brain will push back and trick you into craving for those exact items you were trying to cut back on. I suggest you learn to not stress over the little things. As long as you're consistent, you will begin to see the changes. Instead of beating yourself up, move on and carry on with your healthy lifestyle. One slip up won't ruin all of your hard work, I promise.

Follow Your Budget

In Chapter 2, we will learn that a plant-based diet isn't as expensive as most people think it is, but I imagine you will still have a budget when it comes to grocery shopping. As you go through the store, try to be conscious of where you're spending your money. I suggest you shop the perimeter of the store, as this is where most plant-based foods are going to be. Stick with fresh produce as much as possible, but frozen foods are always a great alternative! Beware of the center aisles as they are typically packed with processed foods. If it's summer, give your farmer's market a visit and support your local food providers. It is a win-win for everyone involved, including the planet!

Remember Your Why

This is very important! At the beginning of any diet, it is very easy to get super pumped up and excited. However, it is normal for people to lose steam along the way. As I've mentioned earlier, a plant-based diet is going to take consistent work. This diet will slowly change into a lifestyle and require you to put in the time and effort day in and day out. So you must continually remind yourself of your "why" and pump yourself up on bad days. Any time you catch yourself slipping just remember why you got started in the first place and it would put you back on track.

Learn to Speak Up

A majority of people do not follow a plant-based diet. In fact, you should go into this journey prepared for eye-rolls and questions from your friends and family. You will probably find this lifestyle even more challenging when you go out to a restaurant. My tip for you is to learn to speak up! You would be surprised to learn just how accommodating restaurants can be or how flexible an item on the menu can become. Of course, I'm not suggesting that you should demand everyone to go above and beyond for your needs, but it doesn't hurt to ask. If all else fails, you can't go wrong with a big salad!

Dining Out

I want you to take a minute and try to answer these 2 questions. First, "how many fast-food restaurants are near to your house right now?"

And second, "how many times a week do you eat at these fast-food joints?" Bearing your answers in mind, one of the most important things I want you to try to do is limit your visits to these fast-food joints as you begin a plant-based diet.

However, if you are invited out for dinner to a fast-food joint or any place where they do not serve any plant-based food at all, the best thing to do is propose an alternative. If that is not possible, simply reject the invitation. Most people say yes to invitations like this out of guilt or the need to please. You should not feel bad if you say "no". However, saying no also requires some grace. Here's a way of rejecting your friends or family without sounding rude – you can say, "thank you for your invite but I'll give it a miss, while it is not something that agrees with my eating habits, please know how grateful I am to be asked." If you face any pushbacks, do not cave. Simply remember your why and stay firm. You could reply to them by saying this – "I'd just rather not but thank you for thinking of me."

Learn to Cook

The easiest and most hassle-free option is definitely to cook your own meals. Therefore, you must brush up on your cooking skills.

For this reason, I've provided you with those delicious recipes in the next chapters for breakfast, lunch, and dinner to help you get started! A plant-based diet is completely doable, but if you're new to cooking,

I suggest that you learn how to cook first. Your food will only taste as good as your ability to prepare them. With a solid cooking foundation, you'll be addicted to whipping up those amazing plant-based delicacies!

Stock Up

If you are looking to set yourself up for success, having a properly stocked pantry is going to be very important. Before you even begin, I suggest getting rid of any processed foods you have. By doing this, you will be getting rid of any temptations. Instead of the Cheetos and Oreos, it is time to stock your pantry with delicious plant-based whole foods.

I find that the best way to go about this is to stay organized! Before you do your grocery shopping, try to get your meal plan together. In the chapter before, I've provided you with a grocery list and a sample meal plan. While this is meant to be a jumping off point, I suggest you start creating a habit of planning your meals every week. This way, you'll be able to get what you need on your grocery runs while keeping your pantry properly stocked!

Support Each Other

When I first started a plant-based diet, only a small group of people supported me. The rest would try to get me to eat ice cream or a double-cheese beef-burger and tell me that I was being ridiculous from "denying" myself these delicious foods. It was hard to be polite and explain to them that I was doing this for my own health and my family's as well. Instead of getting angry and defensive, kindly ask for support instead. If not, there is always an online forum or a Facebook group for you to be a part of. There're plenty of people out there who are going through the same diet and are facing the same challenges as you. When you begin anything in life, a support system is always a great way to stay motivated.

Learn to Read

You know very well by this point that processed foods are going to be a big no-no on a plant-based diet. It will be important to become a master at reading the labels on your food. You may be shocked to learn just how many items contain animal products; this includes your drinks as well! Instead of buying food in packages, I suggest sticking to fresh and whole foods. If a food doesn't have a label, it is most likely whole. Stick with them instead, and you'll be safe.

Learn to Love Vegetables

From now on, vegetables are going to be the star of your meal. Up until now, your vegetables have most likely just been a side dish, but now I want them to take up a majority of your plate. Luckily, veggies come in different colors and flavors, so you'll never bc bored. Build curiosity and love for trying all sorts of vegetables out there because they will provide you with a variety of nutrients that are good for you. If you are struggling to find a vegetable that you truly enjoy, take a few minutes to look at the grocery list provided to you in the previous chapter. I assure you that there is at least one vegetable for every person in your family.

Keep an Open Mind

There might come a time where you'll hit a plateau. There are going to be nights where you don't feel like cooking and get tempted to just order pizza instead, and that is perfectly understandable. When that happens, I invite you to take a deep breath and remember why you started this journey in the first place.

Then, open up your mind and reflect on how the benefits are already reflecting in your quality of life. You've started to sleep more soundly, you've begun losing weight and are feeling more energized. Any time you lose motivation, simply remind yourself of all these benefits you're manifesting in your life. Keep an open mind that more of them will come your way if you just keep putting in the work.

We are finally moving into the final chapter! Here, I'll be giving you my 3 personal secrets to success. Remember, a plant-based diet is so much more than just the foods you are going to enjoy. It is also about living healthier and happier. When you're willing to put in the work, you will experience incredible results.

CHAPTER 2: BENEFITS OF PLANT-BASED DIET

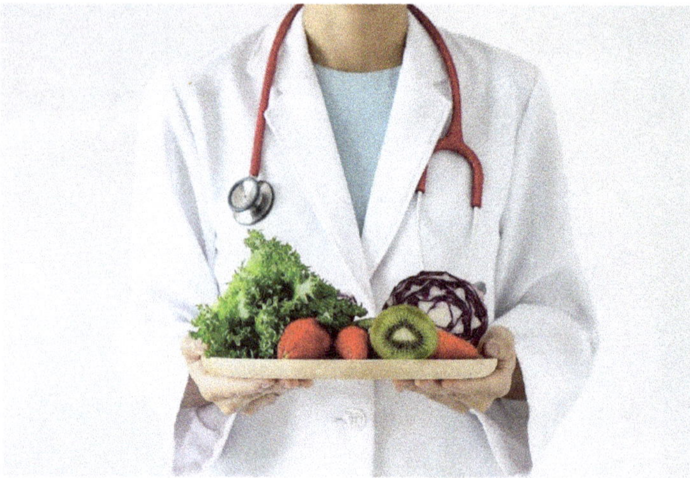

After shifting your diet toward 100% plants, you can attain great overall health along with other protective advantages. There are various protein options available in the plant-based diet as well. In fact, there are many professional athletes and celebrities who follow plant-based eating habits.

Going plant-based is easy, as you can find all products anywhere near your place. At the same time, you save a lot of money, as plant-based food products don't cost as much as the animal-based products.

With that, you can experience all the following benefits:

1. Controlled blood pressure

The immediate and most visible early benefit of this diet is the reduction in blood pressure. People struggle with high levels of blood pressure due to oily, processed animal-based food items. Removing that allows your body to obtain rich potassium content from safer sources.

With potassium obtained from plant-based foods, the blood pressure of your body gets controlled. Balanced blood pressure tends to resolve the problems of anxiety and stress.

There are plenty of plant resources to obtain potassium. Such resources include whole grains, nuts, legumes, seeds, nuts, vegetables, and fruits. Along with potassium, all the given resources also provide a high content of vitamin B6, which also improves the balance of blood sugar in your body.

2. Reduction in cholesterol

One of the biggest benefits plant-based diet offers is the reduction in cholesterol level. Almost every food item from plants contains no or very little cholesterol. Lower cholesterol level in your body saves from heart diseases.

But that lower cholesterol won't be possible if you keep having animal products such as eggs, meat or fish. They all contain a high amount of cholesterol, which ruins the performance capacity of your heart.

3. Balanced blood sugar levels

With sugars absorbed, you don't feel too hungry, which helps your mind and body altogether. Balanced blood sugar keeps your body in optimum health conditions and allows your mind to feel stress-free.

At the same time, you don't eat high-sugar content, which assists in controlling the blood sugar levels.

4. Reduced risk of cancer

Whole foods, low-fat content, and high fiber, all these traits of plant-based foods improve your ability to stay away from cancer. Of course, you have to follow the diet with discipline and also stay away from bad habits of alcohol and smoking.

There are many animal foods that boost the risk of cancer. Breast cancer and colon cancer are two common kinds that have been related to animal-based food items.

Plant-based diet protects you from the risks of animal foods and allows you to live a cancer-free life.

5. Weight loss

If your goal is to lose weight without compromising the nutritional quality of your diet, this eating habit is effective. The guidelines and food options of this diet keep you away from processed sugars and high-fat content.

With that, you can lose weight without compromising your strength or energy. You eat clean and healthy food choices and intake fiber, minerals, and vitamins.

Along with all that, the plant-based diet is also known to make your digestion better. The problem of constipation reduces. Also, the problem of inflammation reduces as well.

All in all, a plant-based diet is an effective way of eating to live a long life without struggling with critical diseases. At the same time, you can eat well and feel the improved strength in your body.

ADAPTING TO THE PLANT BASED DIET

Any change is scary and changing your entire diet can be even scarier. This is why the importance of starting with small changes cannot be stressed enough. Go slow and you will find it easier to adapt to this lifestyle. Don't overexert yourself. The following are some stages that you should follow.

Start By Slowly Cutting Off The Meat - This is a pretty big step and comprises of several small steps. Start off with giving up on meat for one day a week. You could go for something like "Meatless Mondays" and then expand from there. Over time, you can slowly start adding more days of the week to your change plan. Slowly, you would be left with only one day in the week where you are consuming meat.

Another idea you could try is to start off by eliminating red meat from your diet. Give it a month or a couple of months and then move to poultry. After poultry, you could eliminate sea food. Remember to be gradual with the change so as not to overwhelm yourself and your body. Giving up on meat is more of a mental challenge than a physical one and you have to take it slow.

Also, when you have eliminated meat from your diet, you would be filling it up with other things. Most people go for starches, but they do not have much nutrition at all. Instead, you could try to explore different foods and recipes. Dabble with a few cuisines and try plants that you have not tried before. Soon, it would not be a "Meatless Monday" for you but a "Surprise Monday." Instead of dreading the day you cannot eat meat or look forward to that one day you can, you would be happy and excited about trying something new.

Again, this is a judgment call to make the change more exciting and less scary. If you feel that you want to start off by replacing meat with your favorite plant food, then you should go for it. It is all about comfort at this stage.

Eliminate Eggs – Eliminating eggs from your diet is not a difficult step at all. Now that you have cut out the major two – red meat and poultry, you are a Pescatarian (someone who eats seafood but not meat). After you successfully eliminate seafood, you would become a vegetarian. Now, people who still eat dairy and eggs are called "lacto-ovo" vegetarians. After you eliminate eggs, you would have finished a crucial change stage. Most people find this stage to be pretty easy.

Cut Out The Dairy – For many people, this step can be pretty hard because most of us are used to drinking regular milk. However, there are many delicious alternatives to milk and soymilk and almond milk which would only take a few days for you to adjust. The biggest change is the cheese. Cheese is a favorite of many people and of course, it is delicious and might seem impossible to give up.

What you should know is that currently, there are many alternatives to cheese for vegans. Instead of focusing on the things you are giving up, try to focus on the delicious things you are getting to try and taste. Daiya is a good cheese alternative.

Eat Dishes Made of Unprocessed Whole Foods – If you are one of those people who like their veggies, this step would not be problematic at all. However, if you are one in the majority and cannot stand green leafy vegetables, it could take some getting used to. The following are a few examples that are vegan favorites and you should try them out .

• **Tofu Scramble with Veggies** – Organic tofu is high in protein and you need to crumble it for this dish. Stir fry it in olive oil and add loads of veggies like carrots, tomatoes, spinach, mushrooms, garlic and add some spices like sea salt, turmeric, tamari and black pepper (coarse).

• **Steel Cut Oats** – Add some berries, cinnamon, ground flaxseeds and raw nuts to cooked steel cut oats for this dish.

• **Quinoa with Veggie Chili** – You can replace quinoa with brown rice too but the chili is mouthwatering. It consists of black beans, pinto beans, kidney beans, onions, garlic, tomatoes, bell peppers, kale, carrots, tomato sauce, olive oil, chili powder, and pepper and salt.

• **One Pot Meal** – Your one pot meal can have tempeh or its variations, greens, lentils, quinoa and olive oil.

• **Whole Wheat Pasta** – Serve your whole wheat pasta with tomato sauce and oregano, fresh basil, kale, bell peppers, onions, garlic and olive oil for a hearty meal.

• **Salads** – You can go crazy with your fresh veggie salad. Start off with a bed of spinach and kale and add other tasty veggies like mushrooms, carrots, cauliflower, green beans, snow peas, tomato, other beans, nuts, seeds and top it all with some avocado. You can sprinkle the salad with a dressing of balsamic vinegar plus olive oil or olive oil and red wine vinegar.

• **Smoothies** – Smoothies are a way to have a lot of nutrition from a single drink. For the liquid part, you can go for almond milk or soy milk and add frozen berries, flaxseed or chia (ground), greens and spirulina protein powder or hemp.

• **Snacks** – For snacks, it is good to prefer nuts, berries, salads and fruits. You can make some hummus and dip your fresh carrots in it for some added flavor.

Stir fry is a secret every vegan eventually learns and you should know that it makes everything delicious. There are so many meals and combos that can be created from stir fry. Add some veggies to olive oil, proteins, garlic, greens and spices to get a perfect stir fry of your choice. You can try a lot of things and only use veggies that you like. Or, you can go for everything at once and have a great meal.

WHAT TO LOOK OUT FOR WHEN ADOPTING THIS LIFESTYLE

For most people looking to go plant-based, protein is always a major concern. There is this notion that's perpetuated by the mainstream media backed by big meat producers that protein is only found in meat. Well, that's just not true. Traditional staples such as nuts, beans, oats and brown rice come with a lot of protein.

Often, nutrients like calcium are also marketed as coming from only animal-based sources. The truth is that foods like kale, broccoli, and almonds contain lots of calcium. Ask yourself this, if calcium comes from meat, then where did the animal get it from? It's definitely from the greens they eat.

The major concern for most plant-based diet followers is usually vitamin B12. B12, for everyone, is usually found in fortified products, especially cereals and plant-based milk. However, those shouldn't be relied on to get enough of this important vitamin. The best option is to take a liquid or sublingual vitamin B12 supplement simply; just to make sure that there are no issues.

You can adopt a healthy plant-based lifestyle by basing your diet around cooked and raw foods filled with leafy and colorful veggies. These will provide your body with the minerals, vitamins, and antioxidants it needs.

In order to be successful in the beginning stages of a plant-based diet, you must be aware of the array of items that are highly encouraged to consume, especially since we are cutting out or at least minimizing the intake of animal proteins, we need to make sure our bodies are provided with key nutrients.

Legumes and Vegetables

- Lentils: These guys can be pretty simply added to a variety of meals and are loaded with essential protein and fiber, packed into a low-calorie package. In just half a cup there are 9 whopping grams of protein! You can make them as a side dish or use them as a substitute for meat or create delicious dips! Bonus: Great at lowering cholesterol and promoting heart-health!

- Edamame: These delicious cooked soybeans are amazing sources of protein, with 18 grams being packed in just one cup. Opt for purchasing ones with a certified organic seal, since many soybeans within the U.S. are modified genetically.

- Lima Beans: Lima beans offer a great side dish to a variety of main courses or can be added to a hefty salad or soup. They are packed with 7.3 grams of protein per serving! Bonus: They contain an amino acid called leucine, which helps in muscle synthesis.

- Black Beans: These beans are another great multi-use veggie. They are packed with Vitamin B6, potassium, folate, and fiber. Every serving has 7.6 grams of protein. They can easily be used to make yummy veggie burgers, vegan brownies or a killer vegan Mexican meal!

- Chickpeas: Chickpeas are highly versatile and can easily be utilized in a vast array of dishes. They are infamous for making delicious hummus! They are loaded with 6 grams of protein per serving, and they are easy. You can also use chickpea water as an egg replacement known as aquafaba!

- Spinach: Spinach is one of the most superb green veggies out there. Each serving is packed with 3 grams of protein and is a highly encouraged component of the plant-based diet.
- Kale: Kale is the latest superfood of the Vegan world. It is a favorite when deciding to eliminate meat from your diet as it is very high in iron, vitamin K and potassium. It is also extremely high in fiber and vitamin A.
- Broccoli: Once cooked, you receive 2 grams of protein per serving of broccoli, along with a nice helping of fiber.
- Eggplant: Eggplant has a variety of vital vitamins and minerals within it is compound. It is high in folic acid, vitamin C, manganese and vitamin K. It aids weight to lose and cognitive function. Eggplant is a great meat replacement in lasagna!
- Zucchini: This commonly known vegetable (which botanically is considered a fruit), promotes healthy eyes and heart function. They are high in folate and potassium. They are great to use as a substitute for spaghetti/noddles, just grab a spiralizer and get spiralizing!
- Brussels Sprouts: 2 grams of protein per serving is not the only healthy component of this misunderstood vegetable. They also offer consumers a good dose of potassium and Vitamin K.

- Cauliflower: This vegetable is an extremely high source of vitamin A, vitamin B1, B2 and B3. It has even been said that it can be used as a stress reliever!

- Potatoes: Potatoes are a great starchy source of potassium and protein. They are pretty inexpensive if you are one that is watching their budget. Bonus: Very heart-healthy!

Fruits

- Avocado: Avocados are known as miracle fruits in the world of Veganism. They are true super-fruit and incredibly beneficial. They are one of the best things to eat if you are looking to incorporate more fatty acids into your diet. They are also loaded with 20 various minerals and vitamins. Plus, they are easy to incorporate into dishes all throughout the day!

- Grapefruit: Contrary to popular belief, oranges are not your best bet when attempting to add more Vitamin C into your diet. Pick up a grapefruit instead, for they have 50% more than the average orange! Bonus: Assists with arthritis. Double Bonus: Great remedy for oily skin!

- Pineapple: This juicy and delicious fruit can be devoured in an array of ways, which means it is a good item to incorporate into meals. Bonus: Since pineapples are full of anti-inflammatory nutrients, they aid in reducing stroke and heart attacks. Double Bonus: Pineapples have also been known to increase fertility!

- Blueberries: These guys are a delectable treat that is easily incorporated into many dishes. They are packed with antioxidants and Vitamin C. Bonus: Blueberries have been proven to promote eye health and slow macular degeneration.

- Pomegranate: They are filled with antioxidants and potassium. Bonus: Promote heart and cardiovascular health and are known to lower cholesterol.

- Apples: Protect the health of the brain and heart. Double Bonus: Assist in lowering cholesterol. Triple bonus: Aid in weight loss. Quadruple bonus: Aid in oral health. In other words, pick up an apple if you need a snack.

- Kiwi: This tart fruit is loaded with Vitamins E and C, along with many types of antioxidants. They are loaded with fiber and have a low-calorie count, which makes them a guilt-free snack. Bonus: Promote eye health. Double Bonus: Lowers the chances of cancer. Triple Bonus: Aids in weight loss!

- Mango: Mango contains 50% of the daily Vitamin C you should consume which aids in bone and immune health.

- Lemons: Lemons are popularly known as harboring loads of Vitamin C, but are also excellent sources of folate, fiber, and antioxidants. Bonus: Helps lower cholesterol. Double Bonus: Reduces the risk of cancer and high blood pressure.
- Cranberries: Cranberries are known for their levels of Vitamin C, but many do not know that they also a great source of fiber and contain more antioxidants than other fruits and veggies. Bonus: They are a great boost to the immune system. Double Bonus: Promote urinary tract health. Triple Bonus: Assist the body in absorbing magnesium and Vitamins E and K.

Nuts and Seeds

- Peanuts & Peanut Butter: Peanuts are quite an agreeable super-food from the points of view of plant-based and meat-eaters alike. Both peanuts and peanut butter contain 7 grams of protein per serving and can be consumed in a variety of ways. While most types of peanut butter are vegan, make sure to read the label, for some contain honey.
- Chia Seeds: Chia seeds are widely known to the vegan world and can be sprinkled on just about anything and everything. They are an amazing source of calcium, fiber, protein, and Vitamin C. Add them

to your smoothies, breakfast meals and clean eating bowls for an extra bang!

- Pumpkin Seeds: Pumpkin seeds are popularly known as a yummy snack, and can also be easily incorporated into soups, yogurt, salads, and more! They are loaded with iron, Vitamins C, E, and K, and essential omega-3s.

- Almonds: Almonds are commonly used as a substitute for dairy in the vegan world. They are packed with lots of good things, such as B vitamins, iron, potassium, phosphorus, magnesium, protein, and fiber! Bonus: They are known to strengthen bones and lower cholesterol. Double Bonus: They are great for hair and skin!

- Flaxseeds: These guys are awesome add-ins to most plant-based meals since they can be ground up and added to things such as cookies, muffins, bread, cereal, oatmeal, and smoothies. They are packed with B vitamins, zinc, magnesium, and protein. Bonus: They aid in digestion and assist with suppressing appetite, which aids in weight loss!

- Sesame Seeds: Sesame seeds can be easily added to crackers, bread, salads, and stir-fry meals. Bonus: Help in lowering cholesterol and high blood pressure. Double bonus: Help with asthma, arthritis, and migraines!

- Sunflower Seeds: These seeds can be used to make butter, making a great alternative to dairy. They contain B vitamins, iron, Vitamin E, and lots of healthy fats.
- Walnuts: Walnuts have been proven to boost your metabolism, regulate sleep, assist in clear skin, heart function and bone health.
- Cashews: These nuts are low in sodium and are packed with flavor, which is why they are an infamous source of protein and vitamins in Veganism.
- Brazil Nuts: These nuts are high in B vitamin, iron, fiber, and protein.
- Pine Nuts: Pine nuts are low in calories and can be easily paired with many types of dishes. You can bake them into foods or create decadent sauces out of them. They are filled with potassium, magnesium, iron, and many antioxidants.

Whole Grains

- Quinoa: Although it is actually a seed, we treat it mainly as a grain in the way in which it is prepared. This South American gem has an incredible amount of protein and therefore can serve as a great substitute for meat products. Quinoa is an important staple for anyone looking to get the most out of a plant-based diet.

- Wheat: A classic staple, whole wheat is incredibly beneficial to your health. Be sure to steer clear of multigrain, however, and go for the stuff marked 100% whole grain to make sure you are getting exactly what you need!

- Oats: These whole grains are packed full of heart-healthy antioxidants. Oats are great and can be enjoyed as a fulfilling breakfast in the form of oatmeal and they can also be ground up and used as a healthier flour substitute when baking. Unsweetened oats are the best to buy and if you are craving a little something sugary, throw in a few berries or a dollop of honey if you wish.

- Brown Rice: Brown rice is incredibly high in antioxidants and good vitamins. It's relative, 14 white rice is far less beneficial as much of these healthy nutrients get destroyed during the process of milling. You can also opt for red and black rice or wild rice. The meal options for this healthy grain are limitless!

- Rye: Rye is an amazing whole grain that contains four times the fiber of regular whole wheat and gives you almost 50% of day-to-day recommended iron intake. When shopping for rye, however, be sure to look for the whole rye marking as a lot of what is on the market is made with refined flour, thus cutting the benefits in half.

- Barley: This whole grain is a miracle food for lowering high cholesterol. It can be quick-cooked like oats and serves as a delicious side dish. Be sure again to seek out the whole-grain barley as other types may have the bran or germ removed.

- Buckwheat: Buckwheat is a great gluten-free grain option for those with celiac disease or gluten intolerance. It's a great source of magnesium and manganese. Buckwheat is used to make delicious gluten-free pancakes and easily becomes a morning staple!

- Bulgur: This grain is a truly excellent source of iron and magnesium. It also contains a wonderful amount of protein and fiber with one cup containing about 75% of daily recommended fiber and 25% or daily recommended protein. It goes great in salads and soups and is easy to cook. Talk about amazing!

- Couscous: This grain is another great source of fiber. A lot of the couscous you see in the store will be made from refined flour.

- Corn: Whole corn is a fantastic source of phosphorus, magnesium, and B vitamins. It also promotes healthy digestion and contains heart-healthy antioxidants. It is important to seek out organic corn to bypass all of the genetically modified product that is out on the market.

Oils

- Coconut Oil: Coconut oil is full of healthy fats that are absorbed easily in the human body. It is a go-to when it comes to Vegan cooking since it is a great substitute for butter and vegetable oils. It can also be used topically, in treating hair and skin. Bonus: Contains fatty acids that aid in weight loss. Double Bonus: Strengthens the immune system.

- Olive Oil: This oil is the main source of dietary fat in a variety of diets. It contains many vitamins and minerals that play a part in reducing the risk of stroke and lowers cholesterol and high blood pressure and can also aid in weight loss. It is best consumed cold, as when it is heated it can lose some of its nutritive properties (although it is still great to cook with – extra virgin is best), many recommend taking a shot of cold oil olive daily! Bonus: if you don't like the taste or texture add a shot to your smoothie.

- Grape Seed Oil: Formed from the seeds of grapes, its clean and light taste is what makes it a popular component in salad dressings, home-made mayonnaise, and baked goods. Bonus: Great part of a skin and hair beauty regimen.

- Rice Bran Oil: This oil is a popular choice in the Vegan world of cooking, especially when it comes to making stir-fry dishes. It is full of antioxidants and has a significant amount of Vitamin E. It can maintain its nutritive properties even at very high temperatures, which is amazing! Bonus: Rice bran oil has been shown to lower cholesterol. Double Bonus: Has been proven to lower assist with the symptoms of menopause in women.

- Avocado Oil: Avocados themselves are ranked within the top five of the healthiest foods on the planet, so you know that the oil that is produced from them is too. It is loaded with healthy fats and essential fatty acids. Like race bran oil it is perfect to cook with as well! Bonus: Helps in the prevention of diabetes and lowers cholesterol levels.

- Flaxseed Oil: This oil contains omega-3 fatty acids and can aid in weight loss, muscle pain relief, inflammation and prevent premature aging. This oil is not to be used when cooking but can be added to cold beverages such as tea, juice and smoothies.

Herbs and Spices

- Cinnamon: This spice is an absolute powerhouse and is considered one of the healthiest, beneficial spices on the plant. It's widely known for its medicinal properties. This spice is loaded with powerful antioxidants and is popular for its anti-inflammatory properties. It can reduce heart disease and lower blood sugar levels.

- Ginger: Ginger is famous for being not only delicious but extremely healthy as well. It is packed with bioactive compounds and nutrients that make it a great fuel for both your mind and body. It is also known to assist with nausea.

- Turmeric: Turmeric is one of the most nutritional supplements known to mankind. Yellow in color, it is known for treating anti-inflammatory ailments and is loaded with antioxidants that strengthen the brain.

- Basil: A popular choice of seasoning in many types of cooking, basil is best known for its part in Italian cuisine. It aids in anti-inflammatory ailments and is loaded with antibacterial properties, aiding in fending off sickness.

- Sage: Sage is a plant with a well-known aroma. It is packed with bacteria-killing capabilities and is used in many antiseptics.

- Thyme: Thyme is an evergreen shrub that has been utilized both in the culinary arts and medicinally for thousands of years. It's loaded with antioxidants and is known to build the immune system and improve circulation in the body.

- Oregano: Oregano is an herb that has a pleasant aroma, loaded with anti-bacterial properties and antioxidants. It is utilized in flavoring sauces and baked into many types of bread. It's proven to help treat diabetes, cancer, and osteoporosis.

- Chives: Chives are a very nutrient-dense food, meaning they have a low-calorie count but are packed with antioxidants, vitamins, and minerals. Chives have been shown to improve mood.

Now that we've covered some excellent plant-based food items, that should be strongly considered when planning meals, we are ready to dive right in and get cooking. The next few chapters will cover smoothies, clean eating bowls, soup, stews and curries, breakfast, lunch and dinner meals, side dishes and snacks and desserts and treats! Please note: serve quantities listed are based on an average person's consumption, they may vary from individual to individual.

Proteins: they're essential for immunity and muscle mass, and help prevent unhealthy snacking. Protein-rich plant foods include soybeans, tofu, tempeh, quinoa, amaranth, beans, lentils, legumes, grains, seeds, and nuts. You should eat 2-3 servings of protein-rich foods every day. For example, a serving can consist of ½ cup of cooked beans, 1½-2 tablespoons of nut butter, or one ounce of nuts.

Omega-3 fatty acids: they reduce inflammation, triglyceride levels, and depression. Flaxseeds, oil, chia seeds, walnuts, and tofu are excellent sources of Omega-3.

Vitamin B12: is crucial to your health. Vitamin B12 deficiency can cause physical weakness, poor memory, a weaker nervous system, and depression.

Calcium: is very important for your bone health. It also improves the functioning of your heart, nerves, and muscles. Add calcium-fortified tofu, soy milk, roots, legumes, and citrus fruits to your diet.

Iron: is another crucial nutrient. Iron deficiency causes anemia, fatigue, and low immunity. Iron from plant foods isn't easily absorbed by the body. To increase absorption, combine foods containing both iron and vitamin C.

Before you can start cooking, it is important that you clean out your pantry and refill it with plant foods. Get rid of all the animal foods you have, or donate them to relatives, friends, neighbors, or community kitchens.

Foods to Remove from Your Pantry

Enriched bread, tortillas, pancakes, commercial juices, dairy, lard, honey, cottage cheese, paneer, frozen meals, ice-cream, jelly, candy, marshmallows, pop tarts, meat-based sauces, dips, salad dressings, milk, white chocolate, egg-based noodles, pasta, mayonnaise, refried beans, and refined sugar (brown and white).

Foods to Add to Your Grocery List

Vegetables, whole grains, fruits, legumes, nuts, seeds, plant milk, whole grain bread, pasta, pseudo-grains, rice noodles, vegetable broth, vegan pasta sauces, dips, dressings, tofu, tempeh, nut butters, coconut sugar, date sugar, molasses, fruit sorbets, dates, raisins, cornstarch, dark chocolate, vegan vinegars, vegan cheese.

CHAPTER 3: PLANT-BASED BREAKFAST

Pumpkin Chia Smoothie

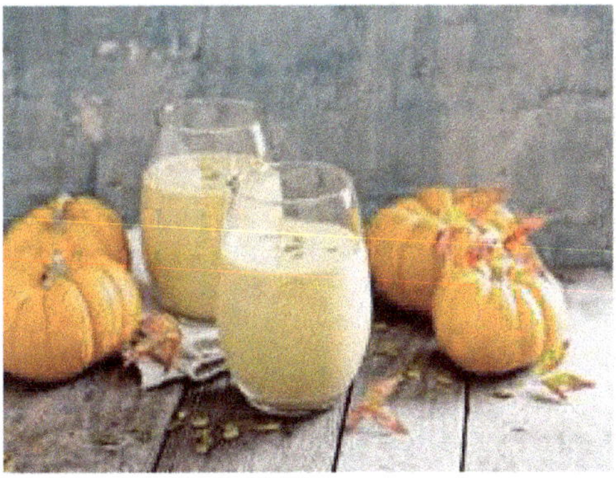

Serves: 1

Time: 5 Minutes

Calories: 726; Protein: 5.5 Grams; Fat: 69.8 Grams; Carbs: 15 Grams

Ingredients:

- 3 Tablespoons Pumpkin Puree
- 1 Tablespoon MCT Oil
- ¾ Cup Coconut Milk, Full Fat
- ½ Avocado, Fresh
- 1 Teaspoon Vanilla, Pure
- ½ Teaspoon Pumpkin Pie Spice

Directions:

1. Combine all ingredients together until blended.

Interesting Facts: Chia seeds are widely known to the vegan world and can be sprinkled on just about anything and everything. They are an amazing source of calcium, fiber, protein, and Vitamin C. Add them to your smoothies, breakfast meals and clean eating bowls for an extra bang!

Cantaloupe Smoothie Bowl

Serves: 2

Time: 5 Minutes

Calories: 135

Protein: 3 Grams

Fat: 1 Gram

Carbs: 32 Grams

Ingredients:

- ¾ Cup carrot Juice
- 4 Cps Cantaloupe, Frozen & Cubed
- Mellon Balls or Berries to Serve
- Pinch Sea Salt

Directions:

1. Blend everything together until smooth.

Interesting Facts: These guys are a delectable treat that is easily incorporated into many dishes. They are packed with antioxidants and Vitamin C. Bonus: Blueberries have been proven to promote eye health and slow macular degeneration.

Berry & Cauliflower Smoothie

Serves: 2

Time: 10 Minutes

Calories: 149

Protein: 3 Grams

Fat: 3 Grams

Carbs: 29 Grams

Ingredients:

- 1 Cup Riced Cauliflower, Frozen
- 1 Cup Banana, Sliced & Frozen
- ½ Cup Mixed Berries, Frozen
- 2 Cups Almond Milk, Unsweetened
- 2 Teaspoons Maple syrup, Pure & Optional

Directions:

1. Blend until mixed well.

Interesting Facts: This vegetable is an extremely high source of vitamin A, vitamin B1, B2 and B3. It has even been said that it can be used as a stress reliever!

Green Mango Smoothie

Serves: 1

Time: 5 Minutes

Calories: 417

Protein: 7.2 Grams

Fat: 2.8 Grams

Carbs: 102.8 Grams

Ingredients:

- 2 Cups Spinach
- 1-2 Cups Coconut Water
- 2 Mangos, Ripe, Peeled & Diced

Directions:

1. Blend everything together until smooth.

Interesting Facts: Mangos contain 50% of the daily Vitamin C you should consume which aid in bone and immune health.

Coconut & Strawberry Smoothie

Serves: 1

Time: 10 Minutes

Calories: 278

Protein: 14 Grams

Fat: 2 Grams

Carbs: 57 Grams

Ingredients:

- 1 Cup Strawberries, Frozen & Thawed Slightly
- 1 Ripe Banana, Sliced & Frozen
- ½ Cup Coconut Milk, Light
- ½ Cup Greek Yogurt, Plain
- 1 Tablespoon Chia Seeds
- 1 Teaspoon Lime juice, Fresh
- 4 Ice Cubes

Directions:

1. Blend everything.

Interesting Facts: Coconut oil is full of healthy fats that are absorbed easily in the human body. It is a go-to when it comes to Vegan cooking since it is a great substitute for butter and vegetable oils. It can also be used topically, in treating hair and skin. Bonus: Contains fatty acids that aid in weight loss. Double Bonus: Strengthens the immune system.

Chia Seed Smoothie

Serves: 3

Time: 5 Minutes

Calories: 477

Protein: 8 Grams

Fat: 29 Grams

Carbs: 57 Grams

Ingredients:

- ¼ Teaspoon Cinnamon
- 1 Tablespoon Ginger, Fresh & Grated
- Pinch Cardamom
- 1 Tablespoon Chia Seeds
- 2 Medjool Dates, Pitted
- 1 Cup Alfalfa Sprouts
- 1 Cup Water
- 1 Banana
- ½ Cup Coconut Milk, Unsweetened

Directions:

1. Blend everything together until smooth.

Interesting Facts: Chia seeds are widely known to the vegan world and can be sprinkled on just about anything and everything. They are an amazing source of calcium, fiber, protein, and Vitamin C. Add them to your smoothies, breakfast meals and clean eating bowls for an extra bang!

Mango Smoothie

Serves: 3

Time: 5 Minutes

Calories: 376

Protein: 5 Grams

Fat: 2 Grams

Carbs: 95 Grams

Ingredients:

- 1 Carrot, Peeled & Chopped
- 1 Cup Strawberries
- 1 Cup Water
- 1 Cup Peaches, Chopped
- 1 Banana, Frozen & sliced
- 1 Cup Mango, Chopped

Directions:

1. Blend everything together until smooth.

Interesting Facts: Mangos contain 50% of the daily Vitamin C you should consume which aid in bone and immune health.

Oatmeal Sponge Cookies

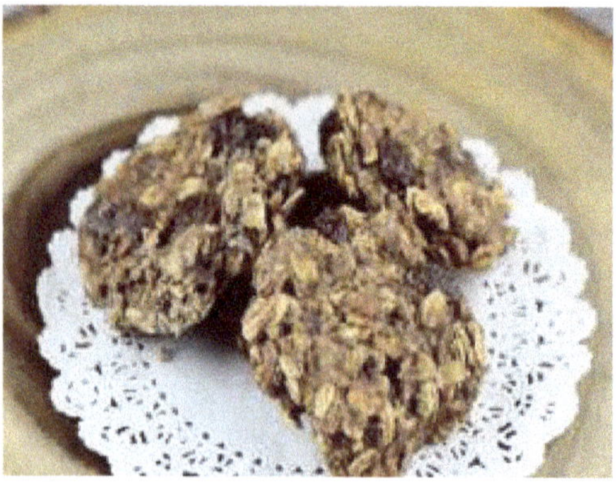

Serves: 12

Time: 25 Minutes

Calories: 79.1; Protein: 2; Grams Fat: 1 Gram; Carbs: 16.4 Grams

Ingredients:

- ¼ Cup Applesauce
- ½ Teaspoon Cinnamon
- 1/3 Cup Raisins
- ½ Teaspoon Vanilla Extract, Pure
- 1 Cup Ripe Banana, Mashed
- 2 Cups Oatmeal

Directions:

1. Start by heating your oven to 350.
2. Mix everything together. It should be gooey.
3. Drop it onto an ungreased baking sheet by the tablespoon, and then flatten.
4. Bake for fifteen minutes.

Interesting Facts: The recipe can reduce heart disease and lower blood sugar levels.

Zucchini Brownies

Serves: 24

Time: 45 Minutes

Calories: 138

Protein: 1.5 Grams

Fat: 4.8 Grams

Carbs: 21.9 Grams

Ingredients:

- 1 ½ Cups Vegan Sugar
- 1 Teaspoon Baking Soda
- 1 Teaspoon Sea Salt, Fine
- ½ Cup Cocoa, Unsweetened
- 2 Tablespoons Vanilla Extract, Pure
- ½ Cup Oil
- 2 Cups Zucchini, Peeled & Grated

Directions:

1. Mix your cocoa, salt, flour, sugar and baking soda together.
2. Add in your oil, vanilla and zucchini, mixing well.
3. Bake at 350 in a nine by thirteen inch pan until done.

Interesting Facts: The recipe is great to use as a substitute for spaghetti/noddles, just grab a spiralizer and get spiralizing!

Vegetable and Tofu with Peanut Sauce

Total Preparation & Cooking time: 30 mins.

Servings: 4

Ingredients:

- 1/3 cup roasted peanuts, dry & chopped
- 8 oz. whole wheat spaghetti, uncooked
- 1 and 1/2 tbsp. soy sauce, low sodium
- 3 tbsp. creamy peanut butter
- 1/4 tsp. red pepper flakes, crushed or 1/4 tsp. hot chili sauce
- 1 tsp. garlic, minced
- 1/4 cup teriyaki sauce, low-sodium
- 2 tbsp. hot water
- 1 bag frozen vegetables (approximately 16 oz. stir fry variety)
- 2 tbsp. soy sauce or 2 tbsp. teriyaki sauce
- 1 extra firm tofu, water-packed (approximately 16 oz. & drained)
- 2 tsp. sesame oil

Directions:

1. Place tofu among some paper towels layers (preferably heavy-duty) and prepare the tofu. Cover tofu with some

more paper towels, pressing occasionally and let the tofu stand approximately 5 minutes.

2. Cut the tofu into ½" cubes and then place the tofu in a bowl. Add either teriyaki sauce or soy sauce, and toss well to coat the tofu completely. Cover; chill for a minimum period of an hour.
3. Cook the pasta according to directions mentioned on the package, omitting fat and salt; drain and keep it aside.
4. Combine hot water, teriyaki sauce, red pepper flakes (or hot Chile sauce), and peanut butter, stirring with a whisk.

5. Over medium-high heat in a large nonstick skillet, heat the sesame oil. Add the minced garlic and sauté approximately a minute.
6. Add the tofu with the pasta and sauté until the tofu has browned a little, approximately 5 minutes.
7. Add the teriyaki sauce mixture & cook approximately 2 to 3 minutes.
8. Add soy sauce, vegetables, and pasta; cook until heated thoroughly, stirring well.
9. Remove the pasta from the heat & sprinkle peanuts over it.

Nutritional Value (Amount Per Serving): 553.6 Calories, 23.3 g Total Fat, 0 mg Cholesterol, 68.7 g Total Carbohydrate, 7.1 g Dietary Fiber, 27.9 g Protein

Breakfast Cereal

Serves: 6

Time: 45 Minutes

Calories: 160

Protein: 3 Grams

Fat: 1.5 Grams

Carbs: 34 Grams

Ingredients:

- ¼ Tablespoon Butter
- 2 ¼ Cups Water
- Honey to Taste
- 1 Teaspoon Cinnamon
- 1 Cup Brown Rice, Uncooked
- ½ Cup Raisins, Seedless

Directions:

1. Start by combining your cinnamon, raisins, rice, and butter in a saucepan before adding in your water. While covered for forty minutes, Fluff with a fork.
2. Serve with honey.

Interesting Facts: This spice is an absolute powerhouse and is considered one of the healthiest, beneficial spices on the plant. It's widely known for its medicinal properties. This spice is loaded with powerful antioxidants and is popular for its anti-inflammatory properties. It can reduce heart disease and lower blood sugar levels.

Fruity Oatmeal

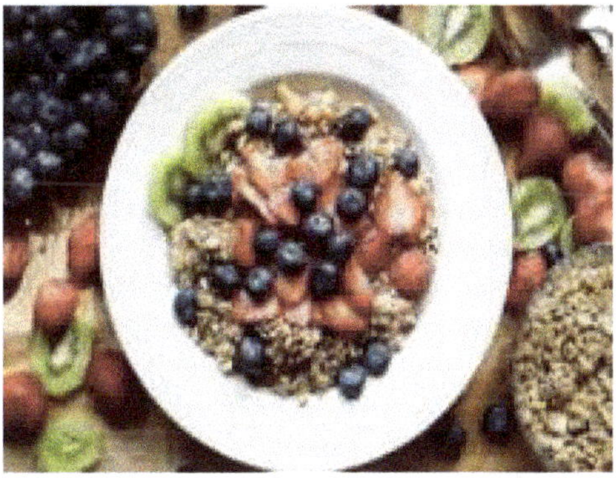

Serves: 2

Time: 25 Minutes

Calories: 230; Protein: 4.6 Grams; Fat: 5.6 Grams; Carbs: 43.8 Grams

Ingredients:

- ½ Cup Apple Juice, Fresh & Frozen
- ½ Cup Oatmeal
- ½ Cup Water
- 3 Prunes, Diced
- 1 Apple, Small & Diced
- 4 Pecans, Diced
- 3 Apricots, Dehydrated, Dried & Diced
- ¼ Teaspoon Cinnamon

Directions:

1. Start by getting out a small saucepan and mix together your apple juice and water, bringing the mixture to a boil.
2. Add a half a cup of oatmeal, cooking for a minute. Add in your pecans, cinnamon and fruit pieces. Make sure to stir. Add in your fruit when your oatmeal is nearly cool.

Granola

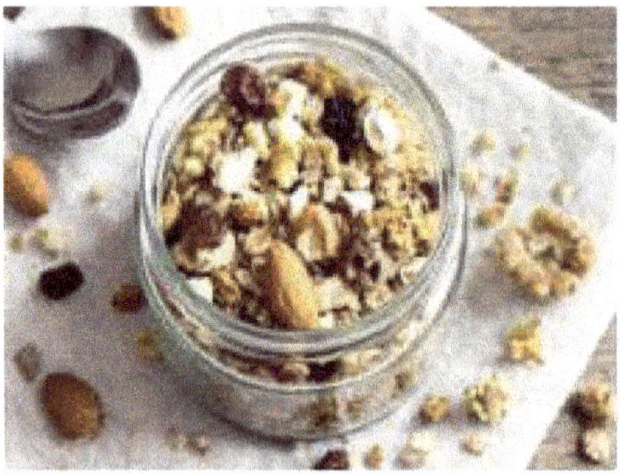

Serves: 7

Time: 1 Hour 30 Minutes

Calories: 239

Protein: 6 Grams

Fat: 11 Grams

Carbs: 32 Grams

Ingredients:

- ½ Cup Maple Syrup, Pure
- ¼ Cup Coconut Oil
- ¾ Cup Coconut, Unsweetened & Shredded
- 1 Cup Almonds, Slivered
- ¾ Teaspoon Sea Salt, Fine
- 5 Cups Rolled Oats

Directions:

1. Start by heating your oven to 250, and then mix all of your ingredients together in a bowl.
2. Spread your granola out over two baking sheets, making sure it's spread out evenly.
3. Bake for an hour and fifteen minutes, but you'll need to stir every twenty minutes.
4. Allow it to cool before serving.

Interesting Facts: Coconut oil is full of healthy fats that are absorbed easily in the human body. It is a go-to when it comes to Vegan cooking since it is a great substitute for butter and vegetable oils. It can also be used topically, in treating hair and skin. Bonus: Contains fatty acids that aid in weight loss. Double Bonus: Strengthens the immune system.

Walnut Porridge

Serves: 2

Time: 25 Minutes

Calories: 312; Protein: 7 Grams; Fat: 18 Grams; Carbs: 35 Grams

Ingredients:

- 1 ½ Cups Water
- ½ Cup Coconut Milk, Unsweetened
- 1 Cup Teff, Whole Grain
- ½ Teaspoon Cardamom, Ground
- 1 Teaspoon Sea Salt, Fine
- ¼ Cup Walnuts, Chopped
- 1 Tablespoon Maple Syrup, Pure

Directions:

1. Start by combining your coconut oil and water, bringing it to a boil before stirring in your teff.
2. Add the cardamom, and then allow it to simmer for twenty minutes.
3. Mix in your walnuts and maple syrup before serving.

Interesting Facts: Walnuts have been proven to boost your metabolism, regulate sleep, assist in clear skin, heart function and bone health.

Avocado & Strawberry Bowl

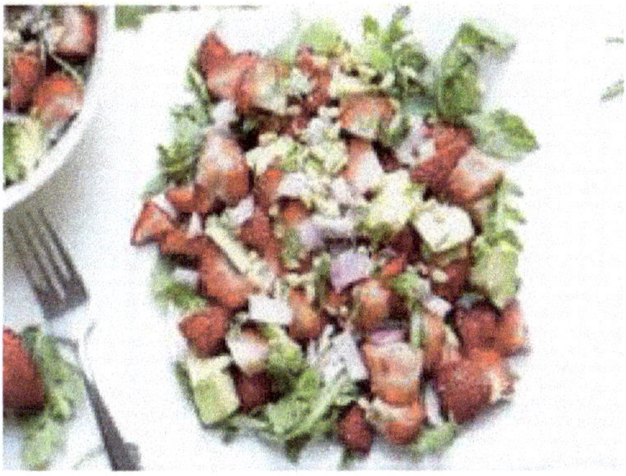

Serves: 1

Calories: 140; Protein: 2 Grams; Fat: 10 Grams; Carbs: 5 Grams

Ingredients:

- 1 Cup Strawberries
- 1 Cup Avocado, Peeled & Pitted
- 1 Teaspoon Lime
- Stevia to Taste
- Pinch Sea Salt

Directions:

1. Blend all ingredients until smooth.

Interesting Facts: Avocados themselves are ranked within the top five of the healthiest foods on the planet, so you know that the oil that is produced from them is too. It is loaded with healthy fats and essential fatty acids. Like race bran oil it is perfect to cook with as well! Bonus: Helps in the prevention of diabetes and lowers cholesterol levels.

CHAPTER 4: PLANT BASED MAIN DISHES

Black Bean Burgers

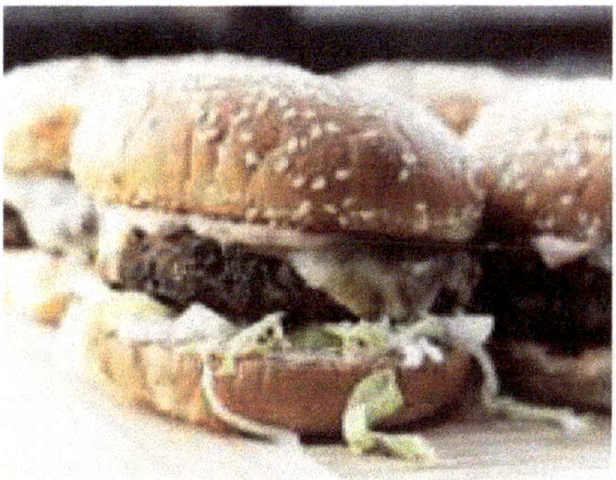

Serves: 6

Time: 25 Minutes

Calories: 173; Protein: 7.3 Grams; Fat: 3.2 Grams; Carbs: 29.7 Grams

Ingredients:

- 1 Onion, Diced
- ½ Cup Corn Nibs
- 2 Cloves Garlic, Minced
- ½ Teaspoon Oregano, Dried
- ½ Cup Flour
- 1 Jalapeno Pepper, Small
- 2 Cups Black Beans, Mashed & Canned

- ¼ Cup Breadcrumbs (Vegan)
- 2 Teaspoons Parsley, Minced
- ¼ Teaspoon Cumin
- 1 Tablespoon Olive Oil
- 2 Teaspoons Chili Powder
- ½ Red Pepper, Diced
- Sea Salt to Taste

Directions:

1. Set your flour on a plate, and then get out your garlic, onion, peppers and oregano, throwing it in a pan. Cook over medium-high heat, and then cook until the onions are translucent. Place the peppers in, and sauté until tender.
2. Cook for two minutes, and then set it to the side.
3. Use a potato masher to mash your black beans, and then stir in the vegetables, cumin, breadcrumbs, parsley, salt and chili powder, and then divide it into six patties.
4. Coat each side, and then cook until it's fried on each side.

Interesting Facts: Potatoes are a great starchy source of potassium and protein. They are pretty inexpensive if you are one that is watching their budget. Bonus: Very heart-healthy!

Dijon Maple Burgers

Serves: 12

Time: 50 Minutes

Calories: 200

Protein: 8 Grams

Fat: 11 Grams

Carbs: 21 Grams

Ingredients:

- 1 Red Bell Pepper
- 19 Ounces Can Chickpeas, Rinsed & Drained
- 1 Cup Almonds, Ground
- 2 Teaspoons Dijon Mustard
- 1 Teaspoon Oregano
- ½ Teaspoon Sage
- 1 Cup Spinach, Fresh
- 1 – ½ Cups Rolled Oats
- 1 Clove Garlic, Pressed
- ½ Lemon, Juiced
- 2 Teaspoons Maple Syrup, Pure

Directions:

1. Get out a baking sheet. Line it with parchment paper.
2. Cut your red pepper in half and then take the seeds out. Place it on your baking sheet, and roast in the oven while you prepare your other ingredients.
3. Process your chickpeas, almonds, mustard and maple syrup together in a food processor.
4. Add in your lemon juice, oregano, sage, garlic and spinach, processing again. Make sure it's combined, but don't puree it.
5. Once your red bell pepper is softened, which should roughly take ten minutes, add this to the processor as well. Add in your oats, mixing well.
6. Form twelve patties, cooking in the oven for a half hour. They should be browned.

Interesting Facts: Spinach is one of the most superb green veggies out there. Each serving is packed with 3 grams of protein and is a highly encouraged component of the plant-based diet.

Spicy Black Bean Burgers

Total Preparation & Cooking time: 25 min.

Servings: 6

Ingredients:

- 1 minced jalapeno pepper, small
- 1/2 cup flour
- 2 minced garlic cloves
- 1/2 tsp. oregano, dried
- 1 diced onion, small
- 1/2 cup corn niblets
- 2 cups mashed black beans, canned
- 1/4 cup breadcrumbs
- 2 tsp. minced parsley (optional)
- 1/4 tsp. cumin
- 1 tbsp. olive oil
- 1/2 diced red pepper, medium
- 2 tsp. chili powder
- 1/2 tsp. salt

Directions:

1. To coat, set aside the flour on a small plate. Sauté the garlic, onion, hot peppers, and oregano in oil on medium-high heat settings in a medium saucepan, until the onions are translucent. Put in the peppers & sauté until pepper is tender, approximately 2 more minutes. Keep it aside.
2. Use a fork or potato masher to mash the black beans in a large bowl. Stir in the vegetables cumin, breadcrumbs, chili powder, parsley and salt. Mix well and divide to make 6 patties.
3. Coat each side of the patty by laying it down in the flour. Cook the patties on a lightly oiled frying pan until browned on either sides or approximately 10 minutes on medium-high heat.

Nutritional Value (Amount Per Serving): 172.4 Calories, 3.2 g Total Fat, 0 mg Cholesterol, 29.7 g Total Carbohydrate, 7.1 g Dietary Fiber, 7.3 g Protein

Mediterranean Wrap

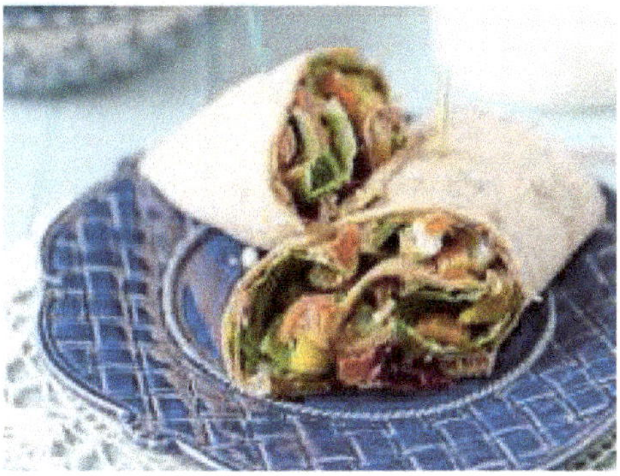

Serves: 1

Time: 10 Minutes

Calories: 428; Protein: 13 Grams; Fat: 23 Grams; Carbs: 47 Grams

Ingredients:

- ¼ Cup Crispy Chickpeas
- ¼ Cup Cherry Tomatoes, Halved
- Handful Baby Spinach
- 2 Romaine Lettuce Leaves for Wrapping
- 2 Tablespoons Lemon Juice, Fresh
- ¼ Cup Hummus
- 2 Tablespoons Kalamata Olives, Quartered

Directions:

1. Mix everything but your lettuce leaves and hummus together.
2. Put your hummus on your lettuce leaves, topping with your chickpea mixture, and then serve immediately.

Interesting Facts: Chickpeas are highly versatile and can easily be utilized in a vast array of dishes. They are infamous for making delicious hummus! They are loaded with 6 grams of protein per serving, and they are easy. You can also use chickpea water as an egg replacement known as aquafaba!

Sushi Bowl

Serves: 1

Time: 40 Minutes

Calories: 467; Protein: 22 Grams; Fat: 20 Grams; Carbs: 56 Grams

Ingredients:

- ½ Cup Edamame Beans, Shelled & Fresh
- ¾ Cup Brown Rice, Cooked
- ½ Cup Spinach, Chopped
- ¼ Cup Bell Pepper, Sliced
- ¼ Cup Avocado, Sliced
- ¼ Cup Cilantro, Fresh & Chopped
- 1 Scallion, Chopped
- ¼ Nori Sheet
- 1-2 Tablespoons Tamari
- 1 Tablespoon Sesame Seeds, Optional

Directions:

1. Steam your edamame beans, and then assemble your edamame, rice, avocado, spinach, cilantro, scallions and bell pepper into a bowl.
2. Cut the nori into ribbons, sprinkling it on top, drizzling with tamari and sesame seeds before serving.

Interesting Facts: Avocados are known as miracle fruits in the world of Veganism. They are true super-fruit and incredibly beneficial. They are one of the best things to eat if you are looking to incorporate more fatty acids in your diet. They are also loaded with 20 various minerals and vitamins. Plus, they are easy to incorporate into dishes all throughout the day!

Cauliflower Steaks

Serves: 4

Time: 30 Minutes

Calories: 167; Protein: 6 Grams; Fat: 13 Grams; Carbs: 10 Grams

Ingredients:

- ¼ Teaspoon Black Pepper
- ½ Teaspoon Sea Salt, Fine
- 1 Tablespoon Olive Oil
- 1 Head Cauliflower, Large
- ¼ Cup Creamy Hummus
- 2 Tablespoons Lemon Sauce
- ½ Cup Peanuts, Crushed (Optional)

Directions:

1. Start by heating your oven to 425.
2. Cut your cauliflower stems, and then remove the leaves. Put the cut side down, and then slice half down the middle. Cut into ¾ inch steaks. If you cut them thinner, they could fall apart.
3. Arrange them in a single layer on a baking sheet, drizzling with oil. Season and bake for twenty to twenty-five minutes. They should be lightly browned and tender.
4. Spread your hummus on the steaks, drizzling with your lemon sauce. Top with peanuts if you're using it.

Interesting Facts: Cauliflower: This vegetable is an extremely high source of vitamin A, vitamin B1, B2 and B3.

Butter Bean Hummus

Serves: 4

Time: 5 Minutes

Calories: 150; Protein: 8 Grams; Fat: 4 Grams; Carbs: 23 Grams

Ingredients:

- 1 Can Butter Beans, Drained & Rinsed
- 4 Sprigs Parsley, Minced
- 1 Tablespoon Olive Oil
- ½ Lemon, Juiced
- 2 Cloves Garlic, Minced
- Sea Salt to Taste

Directions:

1. Blend and serve as a dip with fresh vegetables.

Interesting Facts: This oil is the main source of dietary fat in a variety of diets. It contains many vitamins and minerals that play a part in reducing the risk of stroke and lowers cholesterol and high blood pressure and can also aid in weight loss. It is best consumed cold, as when it is heated it can lose some of its nutritive properties (although it is still great to cook with – extra virgin is best), many recommend taking a shot of cold oil olive daily! Bonus: if you don't like the taste or texture add a shot to your smoothie.

Tofu Poke

Serves: 4

Time: 30 Minutes

Calories: 262

Protein: 16 Grams

Fat: 15 Grams

Carbs: 19 Grams

Ingredients:

- ¾ Cup Scallions, Sliced Thin
- 1 ½ Tablespoons Mirin
- ¼ Cup Tamari
- 1 ½ Tablespoon Dark Sesame Oil, Toasted
- 1 Tablespoon Sesame Seeds, Toasted (Optional)
- 2 Teaspoons Ginger, fresh & Grated
- ½ Teaspoon Red Pepper, crushed
- 12 Ounces Extra Firm Tofu, Drained & Cut into ½ Inch Pieces
- 4 Cups Zucchini Noodles

- 2 Tablespoons Rice Vinegar
- 2 Cups Carrots, Shredded
- 2 Cups Pea Shoots
- ¼ Cup Basil, Fresh & Chopped
- ¼ Cup Peanuts, Toasted & Chopped (Optional)

Directions:

1. Wisk your tamari, mirin, sesame seeds, oil, ginger, red pepper, and scallion greens in a bowl. Set two tablespoons of this sauce aside, and add the tofu to the remaining sauce. Toss to coat.
2. Combine your vinegar and zucchini noodles in a bowl.
3. Divide it between four bowls, topping with tofu, carrots, and a tablespoon of basil and peanuts.
4. Drizzle with sauce before serving.

Interesting Facts: Sesame seeds can be easily added to crackers, bread, salads, and stir-fry meals. Bonus: Help in lowering cholesterol and high blood pressure. Double bonus: Help with asthma, arthritis, and migraines!

Tofu & Asparagus Stir Fry

Serves: 3

Time: 20 Minutes

Calories: 380

Protein: 22 Grams

Fat: 24 Grams

Carbs: 27 Grams

Ingredients:

- 1 Tablespoon Ginger, Peeled & Grated
- 8 Ounces Firm Tofu, Chopped into Slices
- 4 Green Onions, Sliced Thin
- Toasted Sesame Oil to Taste
- 1 Bunch Asparagus, Trimmed & Chopped
- 1 Handful Cashew Nuts, Chopped & Toasted
- 2 Tablespoons Hoisin Sauce
- 1 Lime, Juiced & Zested
- 1 Handful Mint, Fresh & Chopped
- 1 Handful Basil, Fresh & Chopped

- 3 Cloves Garlic, Chopped
- 3 Handfuls Spinach, Chopped
- Pinch Sea Salt

Directions:

1. Get out a wok and heat up your oil. Add in your tofu, cooking for a few minutes.
2. Put your tofu to the side, and then sauté your red pepper flakes, ginger, salt, onions and asparagus for a minute.
3. Mix in your spinach, garlic, and cashews, cooking for another two minutes.
4. Add your tofu back in, and then drizzle in your lime juice, lime zest, hoisin sauce, cooking for another half a minute.
5. Remove it from heat, adding in your mint and basil.

Interesting Facts: Sesame seeds can be easily added to crackers, bread, salads, and stir-fry meals. Bonus: Help in lowering cholesterol and high blood pressure. Double bonus: Help with asthma, arthritis, and migraines!

Tofu Saag

Serves: 6

Time: 50 Minutes

Calories: 210; Protein: 12 Grams; Fat: 13.7 Grams; Carbs: 13 Grams

Ingredients:

- 21 Ounces Water Packed Tofu, Fir & Cubed into 1 Inch Pieces
- 10 Ounces Baby Spinach, Torn
- 2 Tablespoons Canola Oil, Divided
- 10 Ounces Baby Kale, Stemmed
- 1 Teaspoon Cumin
- 1 Teaspoon Fennel
- 8 Green Cardamom Pods
- 6 Whole Cloves
- 3 Red Chilies, Red
- 2 Tablespoon Ginger, Fresh & Minced
- Sea Salt to Tate
- 1 Teaspoon Water
- 1/8 Teaspoon Red Pepper

Directions:

1. Cook your tofu in two batches, making sure to drain it on paper towels. Your tofu should be golden.
2. Get out a Dutch oven and then bring two inches of water to a boil, adding in your kale and spinach. Cover and cook

until wilted. This should take four minutes, and then stir occasionally. Drain well, and reserve the cooking liquid. Place your spinach and kale into a blender, and blend until smooth. Use your cooking liquid as needed to blend.

3. Combine a tablespoon of oil, a teaspoon of cumin seeds, fennel, and red chilies to a skillet. Cook for two minutes until golden brown and fragrant. Make sure to stir frequently.
4. Stir in your ginger, and cook for thirty seconds. Remove your cardamom and cloves, and then discard them.
5. Stir in your spinach, and then add a quarter cup of cooking liquid into a blender, making a puree. Scrape it down, and then put it in the pan. Stir in your salt, and then cook for five more minutes.
6. Put your tofu on top of your spinach mix, and then cover. Cook for another five more minutes.
7. Combine your ghee, cumin, fennel, and remaining red chilies. Before serving add teaspoon of water as you stir.

Interesting Facts: Spinach is one of the most superb green veggies out there. The recipe contains high fiber.

Simple Chili

Serves: 4

Time: 30 Minutes

Calories: 160; Protein: 8 Grams; Fat: 3 Grams; Carbs: 29 Grams

Ingredients:

- 1 Onion, Diced
- 1 Teaspoon Olive Oil
- 3 Cloves Garlic, Minced
- 28 Ounces Tomatoes, Canned
- ¼ Cup Tomato Paste
- 14 Ounces Kidney Beans, Canned, Rinsed & Dried
- 2-3 Teaspoons Chili Powder
- ¼ Cup Cilantro, Fresh (or Parsley)
- ¼ Teaspoon Sea Salt, Fine

Directions:

1. Get out a pot, and sauté your onion and garlic in your oil at the bottom cook for five minutes. Add in your tomato paste, tomatoes, beans, and chili powder. Season with salt.
2. Allow it to simmer for ten to twenty minutes.
3. Garnish with cilantro or parsley to serve.

Interesting Facts: Kidney beans are packed with Vitamin B6, potassium, folate, and fiber. Every serving has 7.6 grams of protein. They can easily be used to make yummy veggie burgers, vegan brownies or a killer vegan Mexican meal!

Stuffed Bell Pepper

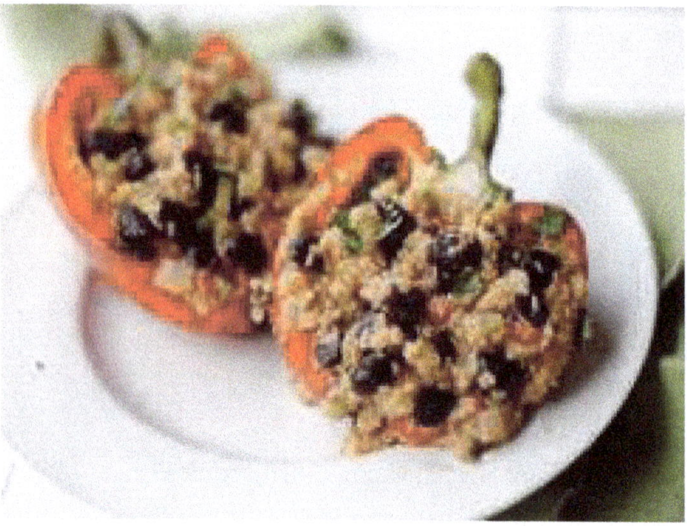

Serves: 4

Time: 25 Minutes

Calories: 126

Protein: 3 Grams

Fat: 5 Grams

Carbs: 19 Grams

Ingredients:

- 4 Bell Peppers, Halved & Hollowed
- ½ Cup Quinoa, Cooked
- 12 Black Olives, Halved
- 1/3 Cup Tomatoes, Sun Dried
- ½ Cup Baby Spinach
- 2 Cloves Garlic, Minced
- Sea Salt & Black Pepper to Taste

Directions:

1. Bake your peppers at 400 for ten minutes, and then mix the rest of your ingredients in a bowl.
2. Stuff your peppers with the quinoa mixture.

Interesting Facts: Quinoa: Although it is actually a seed, we treat it mainly as a grain in the way in which it is prepared. This South American gem has an incredible amount of protein and therefore can serve as a great substitute for meat products. Quinoa is an important staple for anyone looking to get the most out of a plant-based diet.

Ratatouille

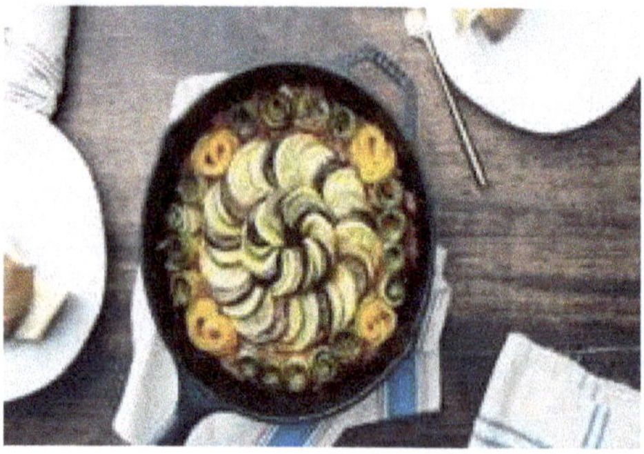

Serves: 10

Time: 1 Hour 15 Minutes

Calories: 90; Protein: 3 Grams; Fat: 25 Grams; Carbs: 13 Grams

Ingredients:

- 2 Tablespoons Olive Oil
- 2 Eggplants, Peeled & Cubed
- 8 Zucchini, Chopped
- 4 Tomatoes, Chopped
- ¼ Cup Basil, Chopped
- 4 Thyme Sprigs
- 2 Yellow Onions, Diced
- 3 Cloves Garlic, Minced
- 3 Bell Peppers, Chopped
- 1 Bay Leaf
- Sea Salt to Taste

Directions:

1. Salt your eggplant and leave it in a strainer.
2. Heat a teaspoon of oil in a Dutch oven, cooking your onions for ten minutes. Season with salt.
3. Mix your peppers in, cooking for five more minutes.
4. Place this mixture in a bowl.
5. Heat your oil and sauté zucchini, sprinkling with salt. Cook for five minutes, and place it in the same bowl.
6. Rinse your eggplant, squeezing the water out, and heat another two teaspoons of oil in your Dutch oven. Cook your eggplant for ten minutes, placing it in your vegetable bowl.
7. Heat the remaining oil and cook your garlic. Add in your tomatoes, thyme sprigs and bay leaves to deglaze the bottom.
8. Toss your vegetables back in, and then bring it to a simmer.
9. Simmer for forty-five minutes, and make sure to stir. Discard your thyme and bay leaf. Mix in your basil and serve warm.

Interesting Facts: Eggplant has a variety of vital vitamins and minerals within it is compound. It is high in folic acid, vitamin C, manganese and vitamin K. It aids weight to lose and cognitive function. Eggplant is a great meat replacement in lasagna!

Cauliflower Rice Tabbouleh

Serves: 4

Time: 20 Minutes

Calories: 220; Protein: 7 Grams; Fat: 15 Grams; Carbs: 20 Grams

Ingredients:

- 4 Cups Cauliflower Rice
- 1 ½ Cups Cherry Tomatoes, Quartered
- 3-4 Tablespoons Olive Oil
- 1 Cup Parsley, Fresh & Chopped
- 1 Cup Mint, Fresh & Chopped
- 1 Cup Snap Peas, Sliced Thin
- 1 Small Cucumber, Cut into ¼ Inch Pieces
- ¼ Cup Scallions, Sliced Thin
- 3-4 Tablespoons Lemon Juice, Fresh
- 1 Teaspoon Sea Salt, Fine
- ½ Teaspoon Black Pepper

Directions:

1. Get out a bowl and combine your cauliflower rice, tomatoes, mint, parsley, cucumbers, scallions and snap peas together. Toss until combined.
2. Add your olive oil and lemon juice before tossing again. Season with salt and pepper.

Interesting Facts: Cauliflower: This vegetable is an extremely high source of vitamin A, vitamin B1, B2 and B3.

Fried Pineapple Rice

Serves: 6

Time: 30 Minutes

Calories: 179; Protein: 3 Grams; Fat: 4.4 Grams; Carbs: 32.6 Grams

Ingredients:

- 2-3 Cups Brown Rice, Cooked & Cooled
- 1 Tablespoon Sesame Oil
- 2 Tablespoons Raisins (Optional)
- 1 Onion, Small & Chopped
- ½ -3/4 Cup Pineapple, Chopped
- 1 Tablespoon Soy Sauce (Or Braggs Liquid Amino)
- ½ Teaspoon Turmeric
- 1 Tomato, Chopped
- 1 Teaspoon Curry Powder
- 2 Tablespoons Cilantro, Fresh & Chopped
- Sea Salt & Black Pepper to Taste

Directions:

1. Start by getting out a saucepan, and then add your sesame oil to the pan. Sauté your onions until they turn translucent.
2. Add in your cooked rice, soy sauce, pineapple, curry powder and turmeric.
3. Mix well and cook for eight to ten minutes.
4. Serve with cilantro, and season with salt and pepper.

Interesting Facts: Pineapple: This juicy and delicious fruit can be devoured in an array of ways, which means it is a good item to incorporate into meals. Bonus: Since pineapples are full of anti-inflammatory nutrients, they aid in reducing stroke and heart attacks. Double Bonus: Pineapples have also been known to increase fertility!

Sesame Bok Choy

Serves: 4

Time: 13 Minutes

Calories: 76; Protein: 4.4 Grams; Fat: 2.7 Grams; Carbs: 9.8 Grams

Ingredients:

- 1 Head Bok Choy
- 1 Teaspoon Canola Oil
- 1/3 Cup Green Onion, Chopped
- 1 Tablespoon Brown Sugar
- 1 ½ Tablespoon Soy Sauce, Light
- 1 Tablespoon Rice Wine
- ½ Teaspoon Ginger, Ground
- 1 Tablespoon Sesame Seeds

Directions:

1. Cut the stems and tops of your bok choy into one inch pieces.
2. Mix together all remaining ingredients in a bowl.
3. Add your bok choy, and top with your dressing.
4. Fry until tender, which should take eight to ten minutes.

Interesting Facts: Sesame seeds can be easily added to crackers, bread, salads, and stir-fry meals. Bonus: Help in lowering cholesterol and high blood pressure. Double bonus: Help with asthma, arthritis, and migraines!

Grilled Eggplant Steaks

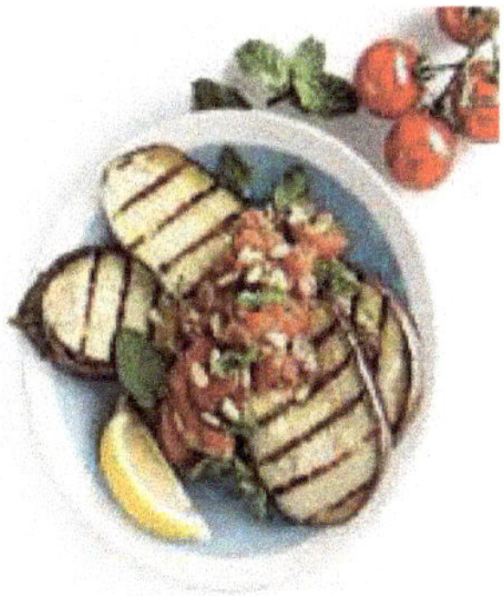

Serves: 6

Time: 35 Minutes

Calories: 86; Protein: 8 Grams; Fat: 7 Grams; Carbs: 12 Grams

Ingredients:

- 4 Roma Tomatoes, Diced
- 8 Ounces Feta, Diced
- 2 Eggplants
- 1 Tablespoon Olive Oil
- 1 Cup Parsley, Chopped
- 1 Cucumber, Diced
- Sea Salt & Black Pepper to Taste

Directions:

1. Slice your eggplants into three thick steaks, and then drizzle with oil. Season then grill for four minutes per side in a pan.
2. Top with the remaining ingredients.

Interesting Facts: Eggplant has a variety of vital vitamins and minerals within it is compound. It is high in folic acid, vitamin C, manganese and vitamin K. It aids weight to lose and cognitive function. Eggplant is a great meat replacement in lasagna!

Pesto & Tomato Quinoa

Serves: 1

Time: 25 Minutes

Calories: 535; Protein: 20 Grams; Fat: 23 Grams; Carbs: 69 Grams

Ingredients:

- 1 Teaspoon Olive Oil
- 1 Cup Onion, Chopped
- 1 Cup Zucchini, Chopped
- 1 Clove Garlic, Minced
- 1 Tomato, Chopped
- Pinch Sea Salt
- 2 Tablespoons Sun Dried Tomatoes, Chopped
- 2-3 Tablespoons Basil Pesto
- 1 Cup Spinach, Chopped
- 2 Cups Quinoa, Cooked
- 1 Tablespoon Nutritional Yeast, Optional

Directions:

1. Heat your oil in a skillet, and sauté your onion over medium-high heat. This should take five minutes, and then add in your garlic, cooking for another minute. Add in your sea salt and zucchini.
2. Cook for about five-minute and then add in your sun dried tomatoes, and mix well.
3. Toss your pesto in, and then mix well.
4. Layer your spinach, quinoa and then zucchini mixture on a plate, topping with nutritional yeast if desired.

Interesting Facts: Quinoa is an important staple for anyone looking to get the most out of a plant-based diet.

Mac & "Cheese"

Serves: 6

Time: 40 Minutes

Calories: 848; Protein: 70 Grams; Fat: 8.4 Grams; Carbs: 140.1 Grams

Ingredients:

- Milk Substitute
- 16 Ounces Elbow Macaroni, Whole Wheat
- 16 Ounces Vegan Mayonnaise
- 3 Cups Nutritional Yeast
- Whole Wheat Bread Crumbs
- Sea Salt & Black Pepper to Taste

Directions:

1. Make your noodles as the package instructs. Drain them, and then add in your ingredients, and mix well.
2. Add in your milk substitute, stirring until creamy.
3. Pour your ingredients into a baking dish and then sprinkle your bread crumbs on top.
4. Bake until it's golden brown, which will take about a half hour.

Interesting Facts: A classic staple, whole wheat is incredibly beneficial to your health. Be sure to steer clear of multigrain, however, and go for the stuff marked 100% whole grain to make sure you are getting exactly what you need!

CHAPTER 5: PLANT-BASED SOUPS AND STEWS

Tomato Gazpacho

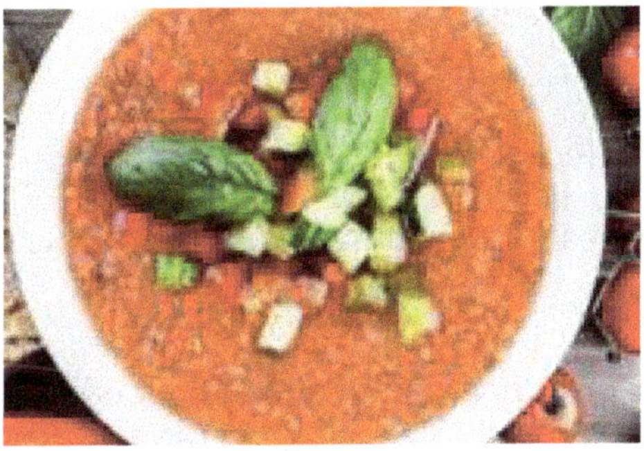

Serves: 6

Time: 2 Hours 25 Minutes

Calories: 181; Protein: 3 Grams; Fat: 14 Grams; Carbs: 14 Grams

Ingredients:

- 2 Tablespoons + 1 Teaspoon Red Wine Vinegar, Divided
- ½ Teaspoon Pepper
- 1 Teaspoon Sea Salt
- 1 Avocado,
- ¼ Cup Basil, Fresh & Chopped
- 3 Tablespoons + 2 Teaspoons Olive Oil, Divided
- 1 Clove Garlic, crushed
- 1 Red Bell Pepper, Sliced & Seeded

- 1 Cucumber, Chunked
- 2 ½ lbs. Large Tomatoes, Cored & Chopped

Directions:

1. Place half of your cucumber, bell pepper, and ¼ cup of each tomato in a bowl, covering. Set it in the fried.
2. Puree your remaining tomatoes, cucumber and bell pepper with garlic, three tablespoons oil, two tablespoons of vinegar, sea salt and black pepper into a blender, blending until smooth. Transfer it to a bowl, and chill for two hours.
3. Chop the avocado, adding it to your chopped vegetables, adding your remaining oil, vinegar, salt, pepper and basil.
4. Ladle your tomato puree mixture into bowls, and serve with chopped vegetables as a salad.

Interesting Facts: Avocados themselves are ranked within the top five of the healthiest foods on the planet, so you know that the oil that is produced from them is too. It is loaded with healthy fats and essential fatty acids. Like race bran oil it is perfect to cook with as well! Bonus: Helps in the prevention of diabetes and lowers cholesterol levels.

Tomato Pumpkin Soup

Total Time: 25 minutes

Serves: 4

Ingredients:

- 2 cups pumpkin, diced
- 1/2 cup tomato, chopped
- 1/2 cup onion, chopped
- 1 1/2 tsp curry powder
- 1/2 tsp paprika
- 2 cups vegetable stock
- 1 tsp olive oil
- 1/2 tsp garlic, minced

Directions:

- In a saucepan, add oil, garlic, and onion and sauté for 3 minutes over medium heat.
- Add remaining ingredients into the saucepan and bring to boil.
- Reduce heat and cover and simmer for 10 minutes.
- Puree the soup using a blender until smooth.
- Stir well and serve warm.

Nutritional Value (Amount per Serving): Calories 70; Fat 2.7 g; Carbohydrates 13.8 g; Sugar 6.3 g; Protein 1.9 g; Cholesterol 0 mg

Cauliflower Spinach Soup

Total Time: 45 minutes

Serves: 5

Ingredients:

- 1/2 cup unsweetened coconut milk
- 5 oz fresh spinach, chopped
- 5 watercress, chopped
- 8 cups vegetable stock
- 1 lb cauliflower, chopped
- Salt

Directions:

- Add stock and cauliflower in a large saucepan and bring to boil over medium heat for 15 minutes.
- Add spinach and watercress and cook for another 10 minutes.
- Remove from heat and puree the soup using a blender until smooth.
- Add coconut milk and stir well. Season with salt.
- Stir well and serve hot.

Nutritional Value (Amount per Serving): Calories 153; Fat 8.3 g; Carbohydrates 8.7 g; Sugar 4.3 g; Protein 11.9 g; Cholesterol 0 mg

Avocado Mint Soup

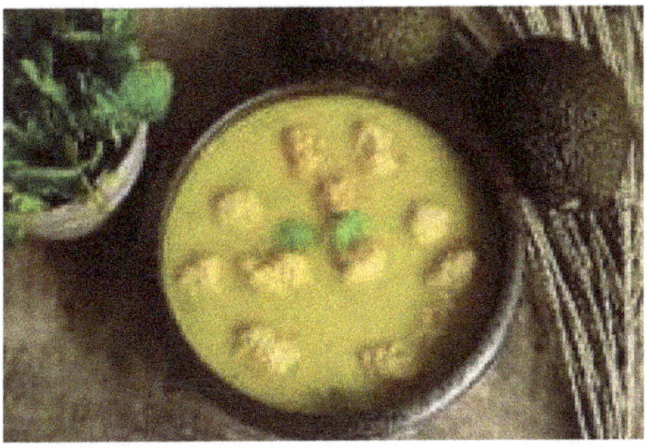

Total Time: 10 minutes

Serves: 2

Ingredients:

- 1 medium avocado, peeled, pitted, and cut into pieces
- 1 cup coconut milk
- 2 romaine lettuce leaves
- 20 fresh mint leaves
- 1 tbsp fresh lime juice
- 1/8 tsp salt

Directions:

- Add all ingredients into the blender and blend until smooth. Soup should be thick not as a puree.
- Pour into the serving bowls and place in the refrigerator for 10 minutes.
- Stir well and serve chilled.

Nutritional Value (Amount per Serving): Calories 268; Fat 25.6 g; Carbohydrates 10.2 g; Sugar 0.6 g; Protein 2.7 g; Cholesterol 0 mg

Creamy Squash Soup

Total Time: 35 minutes

Serves: 8

Ingredients:

- 3 cups butternut squash, chopped
- 1 ½ cups unsweetened coconut milk
- 1 tbsp coconut oil
- 1 tsp dried onion flakes
- 1 tbsp curry powder
- 4 cups water
- 1 garlic clove
- 1 tsp kosher salt

Directions:

- Add squash, coconut oil, onion flakes, curry powder, water, garlic, and salt into a large saucepan. Bring to boil over high heat.
- Turn heat to medium and simmer for 20 minutes.
- Puree the soup using a blender until smooth. Return soup to the saucepan and stir in coconut milk and cook for 2 minutes.
- Stir well and serve hot.

Nutritional Value (Amount per Serving): Calories 146; Fat 12.6 g; Carbohydrates 9.4 g; Sugar 2.8 g; Protein 1.7 g; Cholesterol 0 mg

Zucchini Soup

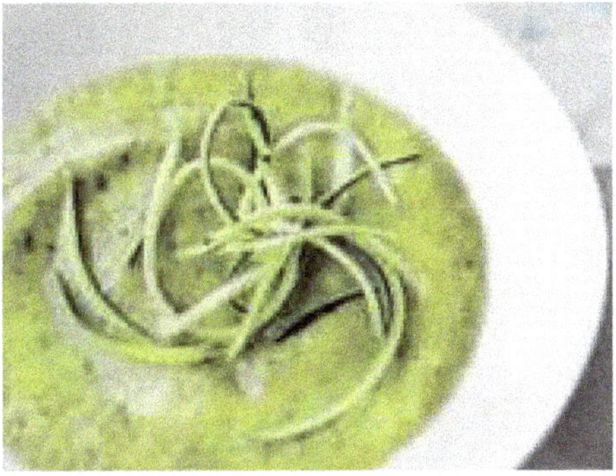

Total Time: 20 minutes

Serves: 8

Ingredients:

- 2 ½ lbs zucchini, peeled and sliced
- 1/3 cup basil leaves
- 4 cups vegetable stock
- 4 garlic cloves, chopped
- 2 tbsp olive oil
- 1 medium onion, diced
- Pepper and Salt

Directions:

- Heat olive oil in a pan over medium-low heat.
- Add zucchini and onion and sauté until softened. Add garlic and sauté for a minute.
- Add vegetable stock and simmer for 15 minutes.
- Remove from heat. Stir in basil and puree the soup using a blender until smooth and creamy. Season with pepper and salt.
- Stir well and serve.

Nutritional Value (Amount per Serving): Calories 62; Fat 4 g; Carbohydrates 6.8 g; Sugar 3.3 g; Protein 2 g; Cholesterol 0 mg

Creamy Celery Soup

Total Time: 40 minutes

Serves: 4

Ingredients:

- 6 cups celery
- ½ tsp dill
- 2 cups water
- 1 cup coconut milk
- 1 onion, chopped
- Pinch of salt

Directions:

- Add all ingredients into the electric pot and stir well.
- Cover electric pot with the lid and select soup setting.
- Release pressure using a quick release method than open the lid.
- Puree the soup using an immersion blender until smooth and creamy.
- Stir well and serve warm.

Nutritional Value (Amount per Serving): Calories 174; Fat 14.6 g; Carbohydrates 10.5 g; Sugar 5.2 g; Protein 2.8 g; Cholesterol 0 mg

Avocado Cucumber Soup

Total Time: 40 minutes

Serves: 3

Ingredients:

- 1 large cucumber, peeled and sliced
- ¾ cup water
- ¼ cup lemon juice
- 2 garlic cloves
- 6 green onion
- 2 avocados, pitted
- ½ tsp black pepper
- ½ tsp pink salt

Directions:

- Add all ingredients into the blender and blend until smooth and creamy.
- Place in refrigerator for 30 minutes.
- Stir well and serve chilled.

Nutritional Value (Amount per Serving): Calories 73; Fat 3.7 g; Carbohydrates 9.2 g; Sugar 2.8 g; Protein 2.2 g; Cholesterol 0 mg

Creamy Garlic Onion Soup

Total Time: 45 minutes

Serves: 4

Ingredients:

- 1 onion, sliced
- 4 cups vegetable stock
- 1 1/2 tbsp olive oil
- 1 shallot, sliced
- 2 garlic clove, chopped
- 1 leek, sliced
- Salt

Directions:

- Add stock and olive oil in a saucepan and bring to boil.
- Add remaining ingredients and stir well.
- Cover and simmer for 25 minutes.
- Puree the soup using an immersion blender until smooth.
- Stir well and serve warm.

Nutritional Value (Amount per Serving): Calories 90; Fat 7.4 g; Carbohydrates 10.1 g; Sugar 4.1 g; Protein 1 g; Cholesterol 0 mg

Avocado Broccoli Soup

Total Time: 25 minutes

Serves: 4

Ingredients:

- 2 cups broccoli florets, chopped
- 5 cups vegetable broth
- 2 avocados, chopped
- Pepper
- Salt

Directions:

- Cook broccoli in boiling water for 5 minutes. Drain well.
- Add broccoli, vegetable broth, avocados, pepper, and salt to the blender and blend until smooth.
- Stir well and serve warm.

Nutritional Value (Amount per Serving): Calories 269; Fat 21.5 g; Carbohydrates 12.8 g; Sugar 2.1 g; Protein 9.2 g; Cholesterol 0 mg

Green Spinach Kale Soup

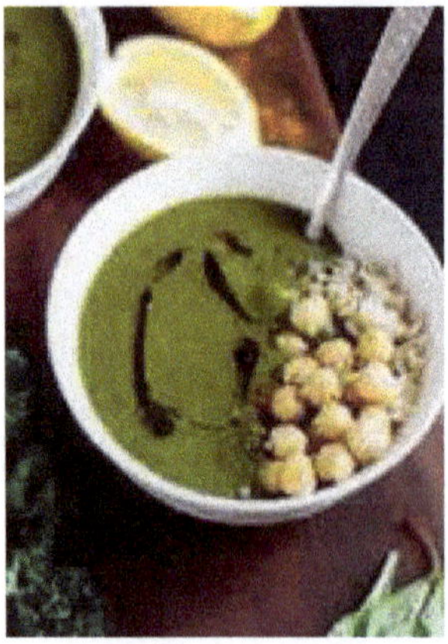

Total Time: 15 minutes

Serves: 6

Ingredients:

- 2 avocados
- 8 oz spinach
- 8 oz kale
- 1 fresh lime juice
- 1 cup water
- 3 1/3 cup coconut milk
- 3 oz olive oil
- 1/4 tsp pepper
- 1 tsp salt

Directions:

- Heat olive oil in a saucepan over medium heat.
- Add kale and spinach to the saucepan and sauté for 2-3 minutes.
- Remove saucepan from heat. Add coconut milk, spices, avocado, and water. Stir well.
- Puree the soup using an immersion blender until smooth and creamy.
- Add fresh lime juice and stir well.
- Serve and enjoy.

Nutritional Value (Amount per Serving):

- Calories 233
- Fat 20 g
- Carbohydrates 12 g
- Sugar 0.5 g
- Protein 4.2 g
- Cholesterol 0 mg

Cauliflower Asparagus Soup

Total Time: 30 minutes

Serves: 4

Ingredients:

- 20 asparagus spears, chopped
- 4 cups vegetable stock
- ½ cauliflower head, chopped
- 2 garlic cloves, chopped
- 1 tbsp coconut oil
- Pepper
- Salt

Directions:

- Heat coconut oil in a large saucepan over medium heat.
- Add garlic and sauté until softened.
- Add cauliflower, vegetable stock, pepper, and salt. Stir well and bring to boil.
- Reduce heat to low and simmer for 20 minutes.
- Add chopped asparagus and cook until softened.
- Puree the soup using an immersion blender until smooth and creamy.
- Stir well and serve warm.

Nutritional Value (Amount per Serving): Calories 74; Fat 5.6 g; Carbohydrates 8.9 g; Sugar 5.1 g; Protein 3.4 g; Cholesterol 2 mg

African Pineapple Peanut Stew

Total Preparation & Cooking time: 30 mins.

Servings: 4

Ingredients:

- 4 cups sliced kale
- 1 cup chopped onion
- 1/2 cup peanut butter
- 1 tbsp. hot pepper sauce or 1 tbsp. Tabasco sauce
- 2 minced garlic cloves
- 1/2 cup chopped cilantro
- 2 cups pineapple, undrained, canned & crushed
- 1 tbsp. vegetable oil

Directions:

1. In a saucepan (preferably covered), sauté the garlic and onions in the oil until the onions are lightly browned, approximately 10 minutes, stirring often.
2. Wash the kale, till the time the onions are sauté.
3. Get rid of the stems. Mound the leaves on a cutting surface & slice crosswise into slices (preferably 1" thick).
4. Now put the pineapple and juice to the onions & bring to a simmer. Stir the kale in, cover and simmer until just tender, stirring frequently, approximately 5 minutes.
5. Mix in the hot pepper sauce, peanut butter & simmer for more 5 minutes.
6. Add salt according to your taste.

Nutritional Value (Amount Per Serving): 382 Calories, 20.3 g Total Fat, 0 mg Cholesterol, 27.6 g Total Carbohydrate, 5 g Dietary Fiber, 11.4 g Protein

Cabbage & Beet Stew

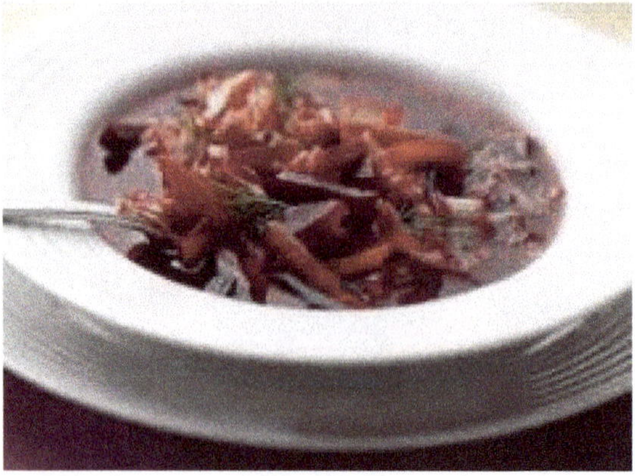

Serves: 4

Time: 30 Minutes

Calories: 95

Protein: 1 Gram

Fat: 7 Grams

Carbs: 10 Grams

Ingredients:

- 2 Tablespoons Olive Oil
- 3 Cups Vegetable Broth
- 2 Tablespoons Lemon Juice, Fresh
- ½ Teaspoon Garlic Powder

- ½ Cup Carrots, Shredded
- 2 Cups Cabbage, Shredded
- 1 Cup Beets, Shredded
- Dill for Garnish
- ½ Teaspoon Onion Powder
- Sea Salt & Black Pepper to Taste

Directions:

1. Heat oil in a pot, and then sauté your vegetables.
2. Pour your broth in, mixing in your seasoning. Simmer until it's cooked through, and then top with dill.

Interesting Facts: This oil is the main source of dietary fat in a variety of diets. It contains many vitamins and minerals that play a part in reducing the risk of stroke and lowers cholesterol and high blood pressure and can also aid in weight loss. It is best consumed cold, as when it is heated it can lose some of its nutritive properties (although it is still great to cook with – extra virgin is best), many recommend taking a shot of cold oil olive daily! Bonus: if you don't like the taste or texture add a shot to your smoothie.

Basil Tomato Soup

Total Time: 20 minutes

Serves: 6

Ingredients:

- 28 oz can tomatoes
- ¼ cup basil pesto
- ¼ tsp dried basil leaves
- 1 tsp apple cider vinegar
- 2 tbsp erythritol
- ¼ tsp garlic powder
- ½ tsp onion powder
- 2 cups water
- 1 ½ tsp kosher salt

Directions:

- Add tomatoes, garlic powder, onion powder, water, and salt in a saucepan.
- Bring to boil over medium heat. Reduce heat and simmer for 2 minutes.
- Remove saucepan from heat and puree the soup using a blender until smooth.
- Stir in pesto, dried basil, vinegar, and erythritol.
- Stir well and serve warm.

Nutritional Value (Amount per Serving): Calories 30; Fat 0 g; Carbohydrates 12.1 g; Sugar 9.6 g; Protein 1.3 g; Cholesterol 0 mg

Ginger Peanut Soup

Total Preparation & Cooking time: 30 mins.

Servings: 6

Ingredients:

- 1 and 1/2 cups chopped cauliflower
- 3 cups water or 3 cups vegetable stock
- 1 and 1/2 cups chopped broccoli
- 3 chopped cloves garlic
- 1 chopped onion, medium
- 5 tbsp. peanut butter, natural-style
- 1 tbsp. ginger, fresh & grated
- 1/4 tsp. cayenne pepper
- 1 can tomatoes, diced (approximately 28 oz.)
- 1/2 tsp. pepper
- 2 tbsp. olive oil
- 1/2 tsp. salt

Directions:

1. On medium heat in a large soup pot, sauté the cauliflower, garlic, broccoli, ginger, onions, cayenne, pepper, and salt in oil until all of the vegetables are tender.
2. Add the peanut butter, stock, and tomatoes.
3. Decrease the heat & simmer approximately 20 to 22 minutes, stirring occasionally.

Nutritional Value (Amount Per Serving): 251.3 Calories, 17.5 g Total Fat, 0 mg Cholesterol, 19.7 g Total Carbohydrate, 5.9 g Dietary Fiber, 9 g Protein

African Vegetable Soup

Total Preparation & Cooking time: 50 mins.

Servings: 6

Ingredients:

- 1 cup chickpeas (cooked or canned)
- 3 tbsp. vegetable oil
- 1 cup finely chopped onion
- 2 diced celery ribs
- 1 potato, small & chopped
- 1/8 tsp. cayenne
- 4 tomatoes, small & chopped
- 1 carrot, small & diced
- 4 cups vegetable stock
- 1 tsp. ground coriander
- 1/2 tsp. cinnamon
- 1 cup tomato juice
- 1 finely chopped zucchini, small
- 1/2 cup crumbled curly vermicelli
- 1 tsp. turmeric
- 1/4 cup lemon juice, fresh
- Pepper and salt, to taste

Directions:

1. Sauté the celery and onions in oil in a soup pot, until onions are translucent.
2. Add the potatoes, carrots, and spices. Cook for additional 5 minutes, stirring over and over again.
3. Mix in the tomato juice, tomatoes and stock. Simmer until the vegetables are just about tender.
4. Add the vermicelli and zucchini and simmer approximately 5 more minutes.
5. Mix in the lemon juice, chick peas, pepper and salt.
6. Garnish with mint leaves, chopped parsley, and strips of pimiento or red bell pepper.

Nutritional Value (Amount Per Serving):

- 172.3 Calories
- 7.6 g Total Fat
- 0 mg Cholesterol
- 24.1 g Carbohydrate
- 4.7 g Dietary Fiber
- 4.2 g Protein

Black Bean and Avocado Soup

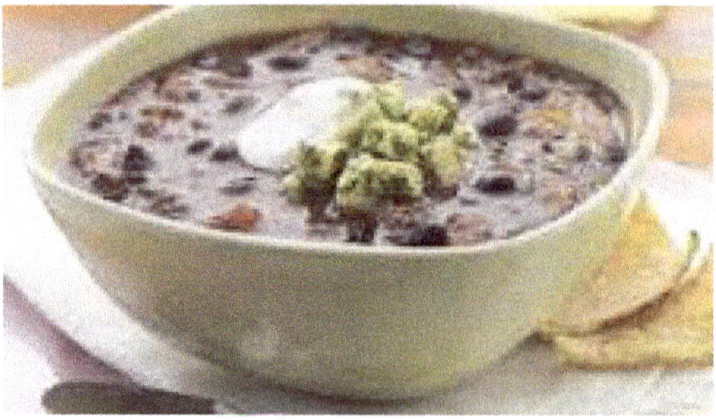

Total Preparation & Cooking time: 35 mins.

Servings: 6

Ingredients:

- 1 to 2 tsp. ground cumin
- 1/4 tsp. ground cinnamon
- 5 garlic cloves, minced
- 1 cup cheddar cheese, shredded
- 1/2 tsp. cayenne powder (to taste)
- 1 tsp. sugar
- 1/4 to 1/2 tsp. salt
- 3 cans black beans, drained (15 oz.)
- 1 red onion, diced

- 1/2 cup cilantro, fresh & chopped
- 6 plum tomatoes, seeded & coarsely chopped
- 2 Hass avocadoes (peeled, pitted & diced)
- 3 to 4 cups vegetable broth
- Juice of fresh lime
- 2 tbsp. olive oil

Directions:

1. Sauté garlic and onion in olive oil in a large soup pot until soft, approximately 7 to 10 minutes.
2. Add cayenne powder, cumin, cinnamon, sugar, cilantro and salt; sauté until very fragrant, for 2 to 3 more minutes, stirring over and over again.
3. Add beans and tomatoes; cook for 2 to 3 more minutes.
4. Now put the broth in the pot & bring to a boil; approximately 15 to 20 minutes, simmer gently.
5. Puree 1 cup of this mixture & return back to the pot.
6. Stir in lime juice, and avocado. Heat through.
7. Place in serving bowls & sprinkle with cheese.

Nutritional Value (Amount Per Serving): 443.9 Calories, 20.7 g Total Fat, 19.8 mg Cholesterol, 48.3 g Total Carbohydrate, 18.5 g Dietary Fiber, 20.4 g Protein

CHAPTER 6: PLANT-BASED SALADS

Cauliflower & Apple Salad

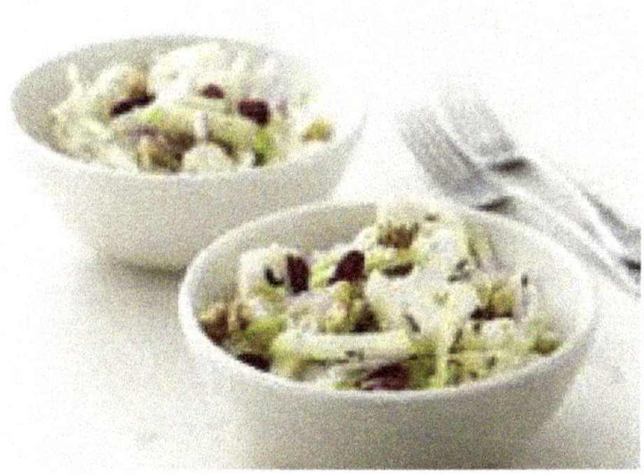

Serves: 4

Time: 25 Minutes

Calories: 198

Protein: 7 Grams

Fat: 8 Grams

Carbs: 32 Grams

Ingredients:

- 3 Cups Cauliflower, Chopped into Florets
- 2 Cups Baby Kale

- 1 Sweet Apple, Cored & Chopped
- ¼ Cup Basil, Fresh & Chopped
- ¼ Cup Mint, Fresh & Chopped
- ¼ Cup Parsley, Fresh & Chopped
- 1/3 Cup Scallions, Sliced Thin
- 2 Tablespoons Yellow Raisins
- 1 Tablespoon Sun Dried Tomatoes, Chopped
- ½ Cup Miso Dressing, Optional
- ¼ Cup Roasted Pumpkin Seeds, Optional

Directions:

1. Combine everything together, tossing before serving.

Interesting Facts: This vegetable is an extremely high source of vitamin A, vitamin B1, B2 and B3.

Corn & Black Bean Salad

Salad: 6

Time: 10 Minutes

Calories: 159

Protein: 6.4 Grams

Fat: 5.6 Grams

Carbs: 23.7 Grams

Ingredients:

- ¼ Cup Cilantro, Fresh & Chopped
- 1 Can Corn, Drained (10 Ounces)
- 1/8 Cup Red Onion, Chopped
- 1 Can Black Beans, Drained (15 Ounces)
- 1 Tomato, Chopped
- 3 Tablespoons Lemon Juice, Fresh
- 2 Tablespoons Olive Oil
- Sea Salt & Black Pepper to Taste

Directions:

1. Mix everything together, and then refrigerate until cool. Serve cold.

Interesting Facts: Whole corn is a fantastic source of phosphorus, magnesium, and B vitamins. It also promotes healthy digestion and contains heart-healthy antioxidants. It is important to seek out organic corn in order to bypass all of the genetically modified product that is out on the market.

Spinach & Orange Salad

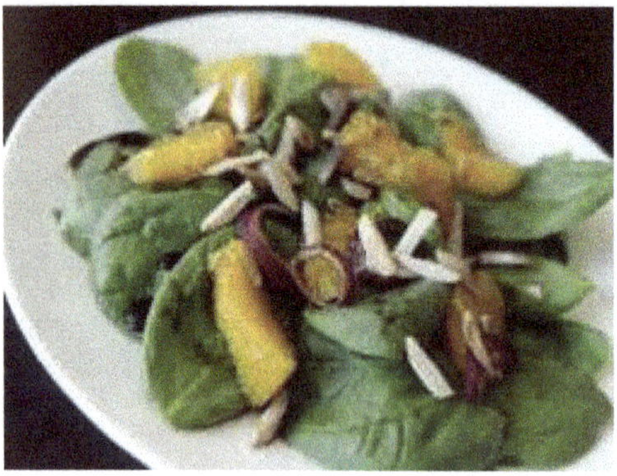

Serves: 6

Time: 15 Minutes

Calories: 99

Protein: 2.5 Grams

Fat: 5 Grams

Carbs: 13.1 Grams

Ingredients:

- ¼ -1/3 Cup Vegan Dressing
- 3 Oranges, Medium, Peeled, Seeded & Sectioned
- ¾ lb. Spinach, Fresh & Torn
- 1 Red Onion, Medium, Sliced & Separated into Rings

Directions:

1. Toss everything together, and serve with dressing.

Interesting Facts: Spinach is one of the most superb green veggies out there. Each serving is packed with 3 grams of protein and is a highly encouraged component of the plant-based diet.

Red Pepper & Broccoli Salad

Serves: 2

Time: 15 Minutes

Calories: 185

Protein: 4 Grams

Fat: 14 Grams

Carbs: 8 Grams

Ingredients:

- Ounces Lettuce Salad Mix
- 1 Head Broccoli, Chopped into Florets
- 1 Red Pepper, Seeded & Chopped

Dressing:

- 3 Tablespoons White Wine Vinegar
- 1 Teaspoon Dijon Mustard
- 1 Clove Garlic, Peeled & Chopped Fine
- ½ Teaspoon Black Pepper
- ½ Teaspoon Sea Salt, Fine
- 2 Tablespoons Olive Oil
- 1 Tablespoon Parsley, Chopped

Directions:

1. In boiling water, drain the broccoli it on a paper towel.
2. Whisk together all dressing ingredients.
3. Toss ingredients together before serving.

Interesting Facts: This oil is the main source of dietary fat in a variety of diets. It contains many vitamins and minerals that play a part in reducing the risk of stroke and lowers cholesterol and high blood pressure and can also aid in weight loss. It is best consumed cold, as when it is heated it can lose some of its nutritive properties (although it is still great to cook with – extra virgin is best), many recommend taking a shot of cold oil olive daily! Bonus: if you don't like the taste or texture add a shot to your smoothie.

Lentil Potato Salad

Serves: 2

Time: 35 Minutes

Calories: 400; Protein: 7 Grams; Fat: 26 Grams; Carbs: 39 Grams

Ingredients:

- ½ Cup Beluga Lentils
- 8 Fingerling Potatoes
- 1 Cup Scallions, Sliced Thin
- ¼ Cup Cherry Tomatoes, Halved
- ¼ Cup Lemon Vinaigrette
- Sea Salt & Black Pepper to Taste

Directions:

1. Bring two cups of water to simmer in a pot, adding your lentils. Cook for twenty to twenty-five minutes, and then drain. Your lentils should be tender.
2. Reduce to a simmer, cooking for fifteen minutes, and then drain. Halve your potatoes once they're cool enough to touch.
3. Put your lentils on a serving plate, and then top with scallions, potatoes and tomatoes. Drizzle with your vinaigrette, and season with salt and pepper.

Interesting Facts: Lemons are popularly known as harboring loads of Vitamin C, but are also excellent sources of folate, fiber, and antioxidants. Bonus: Helps lower cholesterol. Double Bonus: Reduces risk of cancer and high blood pressure.

Black Bean & Corn Salad with Avocado

Total Preparation & Cooking time: 20 mins.

Servings: 6

Ingredients:

- 1 and 1/2 cups corn kernels, cooked & frozen or canned
- 1/2 cup olive oil
- 1 minced clove garlic
- 1/3 cup lime juice, fresh
- 1 avocado (peeled, pitted & diced)
- 1/8 tsp. cayenne pepper
- 2 cans black beans, (approximately 15 oz.)
- 6 thinly sliced green onions
- 1/2 cup chopped cilantro, fresh
- 2 chopped tomatoes
- 1 chopped red bell pepper
- Chili powder
- 1/2 tsp. salt

Directions:

1. In a small jar, place the olive oil, lime juice, garlic, cayenne, and salt.
2. Cover with lid; shake until all the ingredients under the jar are mixed well.
3. Toss the green onions, corn, beans, bell pepper, avocado, tomatoes, and cilantro together in a large bowl or plastic container with a cover.
4. Shake the lime dressing for a second time and transfer it over the salad ingredients.
5. Stir salad to coat the beans and vegetables with the dressing; cover & refrigerate.
6. To blend the flavors completely, let this sit a moment or two.
7. Remove the container from the refrigerator from time to time; turn upside down & back gently a couple of times to reorganize the dressing.

Nutritional Value (Amount Per Serving): 448 Calories, 24.3 g Total Fat, 0 mg Cholesterol, 50.8 g Total Carbohydrate, 14.3 g Dietary Fiber, 13.2 g Protein

Summer Chickpea Salad

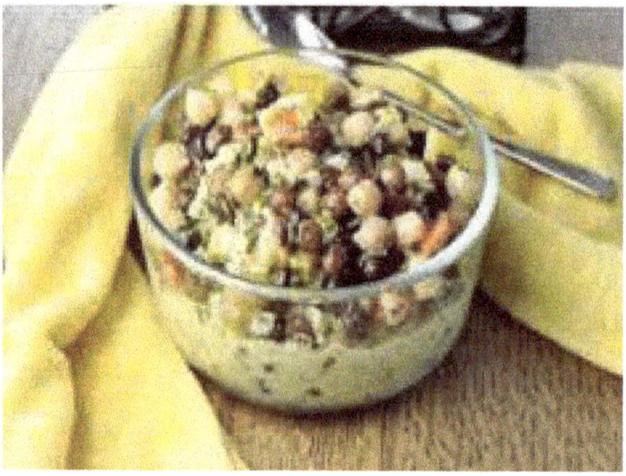

Serves: 4

Time: 15 Minutes

Calories: 145

Protein: 4 Grams

Fat: 7.5 Grams

Carbs: 16 Grams

Ingredients:

- 1 ½ Cups Cherry Tomatoes, Halved
- 1 Cup English Cucumber, Slices
- 1 Cup Chickpeas, Canned, Unsalted, Drained & Rinsed
- ¼ Cup Red Onion, Slivered

- 2 Tablespoon Olive Oil
- 1 ½ Tablespoons Lemon Juice, Fresh
- 1 ½ Tablespoons Lemon Juice, Fresh
- Sea Salt & Black Pepper to Taste

Directions:

1. Mix everything together, and toss to combine before serving.

Interesting Facts: Chickpeas are highly versatile and can easily be utilized in a vast array of dishes. They are infamous for making delicious hummus! They are loaded with 6 grams of protein per serving, and they are easy. You can also use chickpea water as an egg replacement known as aquafaba!

Edamame Salad

Serves: 1

Time: 15 Minutes

Calories: 299; Protein: 20 Grams; Fat: 9 Grams; Carbs: 38 Grams

Ingredients:

- ¼ Cup Red Onion, Chopped
- 1 Cup Corn Kernels, Fresh
- 1 Cup Edamame Beans, Shelled & Thawed
- 1 Red Bell Pepper, Chopped
- 2-3 Tablespoons Lime Juice, Fresh
- 5-6 Basil Leaves, Fresh & Sliced
- 5-6 Mint Leaves, Fresh & Sliced
- Sea Salt & Black Pepper to Taste

Directions:

1. Place everything into a Mason jar, and then seal the jar tightly. Shake well before serving.

Interesting Facts: Whole corn is a fantastic source of phosphorus, magnesium, and B vitamins. It also promotes healthy digestion and contains heart-healthy antioxidants. It is important to seek out organic corn in order to bypass all of the genetically modified product that is out on the market.

Fruity Kale Salad

Serves: 4

Time: 30 Minutes

Calories: 220; Protein: 4 Grams; Fat: 17 Grams; Carbs: 16 Grams

Ingredients:

Salad:

- 10 Ounces Baby Kale
- ½ Cup Pomegranate Arils
- 1 Tablespoon Olive Oil
- 1 Apple, Sliced

Dressing:

- 3 Tablespoons Apple Cider Vinegar
- 3 Tablespoons Olive Oil
- 1 Tablespoon Tahini Sauce (Optional)
- Sea Salt & Black Pepper to Taste

Directions:

1. Wash and dry the kale. If kale is too expensive, you can also use lettuce, arugula or spinach. Take the stems out, and chop it.
2. Combine all of your salad ingredients together.
3. Combine all of your dressing ingredients together before drizzling it over the salad to serve.

Interesting Facts: Kale is the latest superfood of the Vegan world. It is a favorite when deciding to eliminate meat from your diet, as it is very high in iron, vitamin K and potassium. It is also extremely high in fiber and vitamin A.

Olive & Fennel Salad

Serves: 3

Time: 5 Minutes

Calories: 331; Protein: 3 Grams; Fat: 29 Grams; Carbs: 15 Grams

Ingredients:

- 6 Tablespoons Olive Oil
- 3 Fennel Bulbs, Trimmed, Cored & Quartered
- 2 Tablespoons Parsley, Fresh & Chopped
- 1 Lemon, Juiced & Zested
- 12 Black Olives
- Sea Salt & Black Pepper to Taste

Directions:

1. Grease your baking dish, and then place your fennel in it. Make sure the cut side is up.
2. Mix your lemon zest, lemon juice, salt, pepper and oil, pouring it over your fennel.
3. Sprinkle your olives over it, and bake at 400.
4. Serve with parsley.

Interesting Facts: This oil is the main source of dietary fat in a variety of diets. It contains many vitamins and minerals that play a part in reducing the risk of stroke and lowers cholesterol and high blood pressure and can also aid in weight loss. It is best consumed cold, as when it is heated it can lose some of its nutritive properties (although it is still great to cook with – extra virgin is best), many recommend taking a shot of cold oil olive daily! Bonus: if you don't like the taste or texture add a shot to your smoothie.

Avocado & Radish Salad

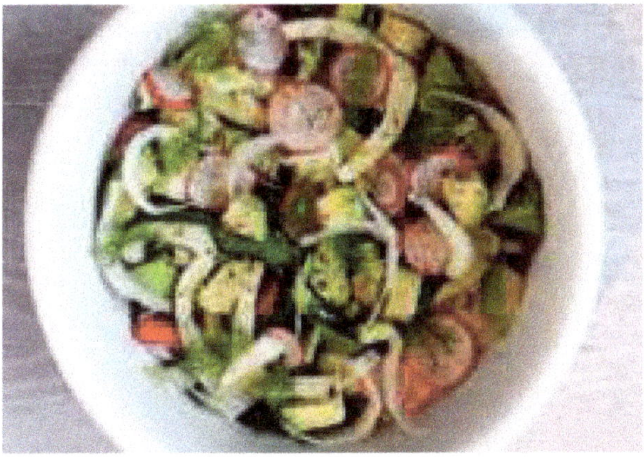

Serves: 2

Time: 10 Minutes

Calories: 223

Protein: 3 Grams

Fat: 19 Grams

Carbs: 10 Grams

Ingredients:

- 1 Avocado, Sliced
- 6 Radishes, Sliced
- 2 Tomatoes, Sliced
- 1 Lettuce Head, Leaves Separated
- ½ Red Onion, Peeled & Sliced

Dressing:

- ½ Cup Olive Oil
- ¼ Cup Lime Juice, Fresh
- ¼ Cup Apple Cider Vinegar
- 3 Cloves Garlic, Chopped Fine
- Sea Salt & Black Pepper to Taste

Directions:

1. Spread your lettuce leaves on a platter, and then layer with your onion, tomatoes, avocado and radishes.
2. Whisk your dressing ingredients together before drizzling it over your salad.

Interesting Facts: Avocados themselves are ranked within the top five of the healthiest foods on the planet, so you know that the oil that is produced from them is too. It is loaded with healthy fats and essential fatty acids. Like race bran oil it is perfect to cook with as well! Bonus: Helps in the prevention of diabetes and lowers cholesterol levels.

Zucchini & Lemon Salad

Serves: 2

Time: 3 Hours 10 Minutes

Calories: 159

Protein: 3 g

Fat: 14 g

Net Carbs: 7 g

Ingredients:

- 1 Green Zucchini, Sliced into Rounds
- 1 Yellow Squash, Zucchini, Sliced into Rounds
- 1 Clove Garlic, Peeled & Chopped
- 2 Tablespoons Olive Oil
- 2 Tablespoons Basil, Fresh
- 1 Lemon, Juiced & Zested
- ¼ Cup Coconut Milk
- Sea Salt & Black Pepper to Taste

Directions:

1. Refrigerate all ingredients for three hours before serving.

Interesting Facts: Lemons are popularly known as harboring loads of Vitamin C, but are also excellent sources of folate, fiber, and antioxidants. Bonus: Helps lower cholesterol. Double Bonus: Reduces risk of cancer and high blood pressure.

Watercress & Blood Orange Salad

Serves: 4

Time: 10 Minutes

Calories: 94; Protein: 2 g; Fat: 5 g; Carbs: 13 g

Ingredients:

- 1 Tablespoon Hazelnuts, Toasted & Chopped
- 2 Blood Oranges (or Navel Oranges)
- 3 Cups watercress, Stems Removed
- 1/8 Teaspoon Sea Salt, Fine
- 1 Tablespoon Lemon Juice, Fresh
- 1 Tablespoon Honey, Raw
- 1 Tablespoon Water
- 2 Tablespoons Chives, Fresh

Directions:

1. Whisk your oil, honey, lemon juice, chives, salt and water together. Add in your watercress, tossing until it's coated.
2. Arrange the mixture onto salad plates, and top with orange slices. Drizzle with remaining liquid, and sprinkle with hazelnuts.

Interesting Facts: Lemons are popularly known as harboring loads of Vitamin C, but are also excellent sources of folate, fiber, and antioxidants. Bonus: Helps lower cholesterol. Double Bonus: Reduces risk of cancer and high blood pressure.

Parsley Salad

Serves: 8

Time: 30 Minutes

Calories: 165.2; Protein: 3.8g; Fat: 9.1 g; Carbs: 20.1 g

Ingredients:

- 3 Lemons, Juiced
- 150 Grams Flat Lea Parsley, Chopped Fine
- 1 Cup Boiled Water
- 5 Tablespoons Olive Oil
- Sea Salt & Black Pepper to Taste
- 6 Green Onions, Chopped Fine
- 1 Cup Bulgur
- 4 Tomatoes, Chopped Fine

Directions:

1. Add your Bulgur to your water, and mix well. Put a towel on top of it to steam it. Keep it to the side, and then chop your spring onions, tomatoes and parsley. Put them in your salad bowl.
2. Pour your juice into the mixture, and then add in your olive oil, salt and pepper.
3. Put this mixture over your bulgur to serve.

Tomato Eggplant Spinach Salad

Total Time: 30 minutes

Serves: 4

Calories: 163; Protein 2 g; Fat: 13 g; Carbs: 10 g; Sugar: 3 g

Ingredients:

- 1 large eggplant, cut into 3/4 inch slices
- 5 oz spinach
- 1 tbsp sun-dried tomatoes, chopped
- 1 tbsp oregano, chopped
- 1 tbsp parsley, chopped
- 1 tbsp fresh mint, chopped
- 1 tbsp shallot, chopped
- For dressing:
- 1/4 cup olive oil
- 1/2 lemon juice
- 1/2 tsp smoked paprika
- 1 tsp Dijon mustard
- 1 tsp tahini
- 2 garlic cloves, minced
- Pepper
- Salt

Directions:

- Place sliced eggplants into the large bowl and sprinkle with salt and set aside for minutes.
- In a small bowl mix together all dressing ingredients. Set aside.
- Heat grill to medium-high heat.
- In a large bowl, add shallot, sun-dried tomatoes, herbs, and spinach.
- Rinse eggplant slices and pat dry with paper towel.
- Brush eggplant slices with olive oil and grill on medium high heat for 3-4 minutes on each side.
- Let cool the grilled eggplant slices then cut into quarters.
- Add eggplant to the salad bowl and pour dressing over salad. Toss well.
- Serve and enjoy.

Cauliflower Radish Salad

Total Time: 15 minutes

Serves: 4

Calories: 58; Protein: 2.1 g; Fat: 3.8 g; Carbs: 5.6 g; Sugar: 2.1 g

Ingredients:

- 12 radishes, trimmed and chopped
- 1 tsp dried dill
- 1 tsp Dijon mustard
- 1 tbsp cider vinegar
- 1 tbsp olive oil
- 1 cup parsley, chopped
- ½ medium cauliflower head, trimmed and chopped
- ½ tsp black pepper
- ¼ tsp sea salt

Directions:

- In a mixing bowl, combine together cauliflower, parsley, and radishes.
- In a small bowl, whisk together olive oil, dill, mustard, vinegar, pepper, and salt.
- Pour dressing over salad and toss well.
- Serve immediately and enjoy.

Celery Salad

Total Time: 10 minutes

Serves: 6

Calories: 38; Protein: 0.8 g; Fat: 2.5 g; Carbs: 3.3 g; Sugar: 1.5 g

Ingredients:

- 6 cups celery, sliced
- ¼ tsp celery seed
- 1 tbsp lemon juice
- 2 tsp lemon zest, grated
- 1 tbsp parsley, chopped
- 1 tbsp olive oil
- Sea salt

Directions:

- Add all ingredients into the large mixing bowl and toss well.
- Serve immediately and enjoy.

CHAPTER 7: PLANT-BASED SNACKS

Radish Chips

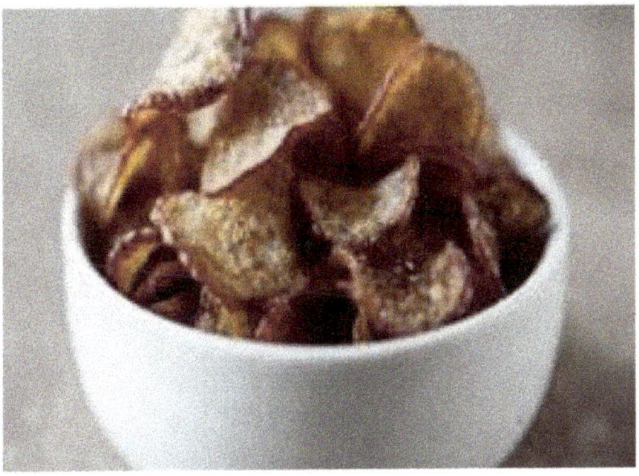

Serves: 4

Time: 20 Minutes

Calories: 3.6; Protein: 0.2 Grams; Fat: 0 Grams; Carbs: 0.8 Grams

Ingredients:

- 10-15 Radishes, Large
- Sea Salt & Black Pepper to Taste

Directions:

1. Start by heating your oven to 375.
2. Slice your radishes thin, and then spread them out on a cookie sheet that's been sprayed with cooking spray.
3. Mist the radishes with cooking spray, and then season with salt and pepper.
4. Bake for ten minutes, and then flip.
5. Bake for five to ten minutes more. They should be crispy.

Interesting Facts: Potatoes are a great starchy source of potassium and protein. They are pretty inexpensive if you are one that is watching their budget.

Kale Chips

Serves: 4

Time: 25 Minutes

Calories: 25.1; Protein: 1.7 Grams; Fat: 0.4 Grams; Carbs: 5 Grams

Ingredients:

- 1 Bunch Kale
- 1 Spritz Olive Oil

Directions:

1. Heat your oven to 250, and then wash your kale before patting it dry.
2. Arrange your kale on a prepared baking sheet, making sure your kale doesn't overlap. Spray it down with olive oil, and then season with salt.
3. Cook for twenty minutes.

Interesting Facts: Kale is the latest superfood of the Vegan world. It is a favorite when deciding to eliminate meat from your diet as it is very high in iron, vitamin K and potassium.

Beetroot and Mustard Chips

(Prep time: 45 minutes/4 Servings)

Ingredients:

- 5 beets
- 2 tablespoons olive oil
- 2 pinches ground mustard seeds
- Salt and pepper to taste

Instructions:

1. Preheat oven to 400□F. Grease 2 baking sheets with olive oil.
2. Peel and slice the beets thinly using a mandolin, or the wide angle on a (cheese) grater.
3. Place the beets in a bowl. Toss with olive oil. Season with mustard seeds, salt and pepper.
4. Arrange beets in a single layer on baking sheets. Bake 40 minutes, or until crispy.
5. Cool for 5 minutes before serving.

Nutritional Values:

- Carbohydrates: 10.4 grams
- Fat: 7.1 grams
- Protein: 1.8 grams

Roasted Kale Chips

(Prep time: 20 minutes/3 Servings)

Ingredients:

- 3 cups chopped kale, de-stemmed
- 2 tablespoons of extra virgin olive oil
- Salt and pepper to taste

Instructions:

1. Preheat the oven to 400□F. Line a baking tray with parchment paper.
2. Place the kale in a large bowl. Drizzle with olive oil. Season with salt and pepper.
3. Arrange the kale in a single layer on baking tray.
4. Bake for 12 minutes or until they become crispy.
5. Serve hot or cold.

Nutritional Values:

- Carbohydrates: 10 grams
- Fat: 3.9 grams
- Protein: 2.5 grams

Pumpkin & Cinnamon Fudge

Serves: 25

Time: 2 Hours 10 Minutes

Calories: 110; Protein: 1.2 Grams; Fat: 10.63 Grams; Carbs: 5 Grams

Ingredients:

- 1 Teaspoon Ground Cinnamon
- 1 Cup Pumpkin Puree
- ¼ Teaspoon Nutmeg, Ground
- 1 ¾ Cup Coconut Butter, Melted
- 1 Tablespoon Coconut Oil

Directions:

1. Mix together your pumpkin, spices, coconut butter and coconut oil, whisking together.
2. Spread this mixture into a pan, and then cover it with foil. Press it down, and then discard the foil.
3. Refrigerate for two hours, and then chop into squares.

Interesting Facts: The recipe is loaded with iron, Vitamins C, E, and K, and essential omega-3s.

Black Bean Dip

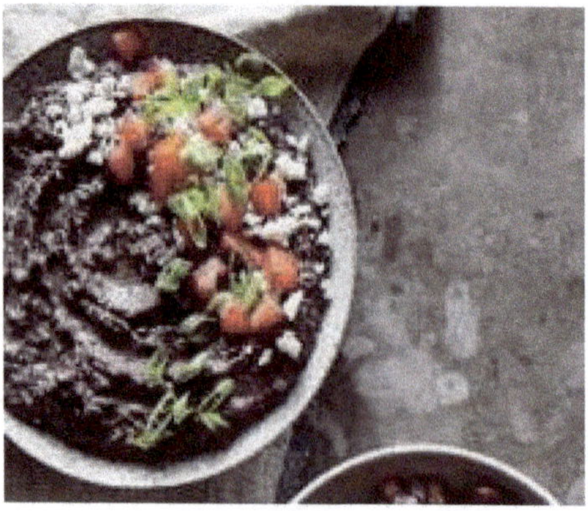

Serves: 2

Time: 10 Minutes

Calories: 190; Protein: 13 Grams; Fat: 1 Gram; Carbs: 35 Grams

Ingredients:

- 14 Ounces Black Beans, Drained & Rinsed
- 1 Lime, Juiced & Zested
- ¼ Cup Cilantro, Fresh & Chopped
- ¼ Cup Water
- 1 Teaspoon Cumin
- 1 Tablespoon Tamari
- Pinch Cayenne Pepper

Directions:

1. Process everything but your cilantro together until smooth, and then serve garnished with cilantro.

Interesting Facts: The recipe aid in digestion and assist with suppressing appetite, which aids in weight loss!

Vegan Nacho Cheese Sauce

Total Preparation & Cooking time: 30 mins.

Servings: 20

Ingredients:

- 3 1/2 cups water
- Juice of 2 lemons
- 2 cups cashews, raw
- 1 tsp. garlic powder
- 3/4 tsp. paprika
- 1 tsp. onion powder
- 1/2 cup nutritional yeast
- 1 can pimientos (7 oz. and include the liquid)
- 3 tsp. salt

Directions:

1. Soak the raw cashews for couple of hours.
2. Put all of the ingredients with 2 and 1/2 cups of water into a blender & blend until smooth.
3. Transfer the blended mixture to a saucepan & add the left over water.
4. In a saucepan, heat the mixture approximately 20 minutes.
5. To prevent it from burning, stir continually.
6. If required, put more quantity of water to your desired consistency.
7. Use as a replacement for cheese or as a nacho cheese dip!

Nutritional Value (Amount Per Serving): 98.8 Calories, 6.8 g Total Fat, 0 mg Cholesterol, 7.6 g Total Carbohydrate, 2 g Dietary Fiber, 4.2g Protein

CHAPTER 8: PLANT-BASED DESSERT

Pecan & Blueberry Crumble

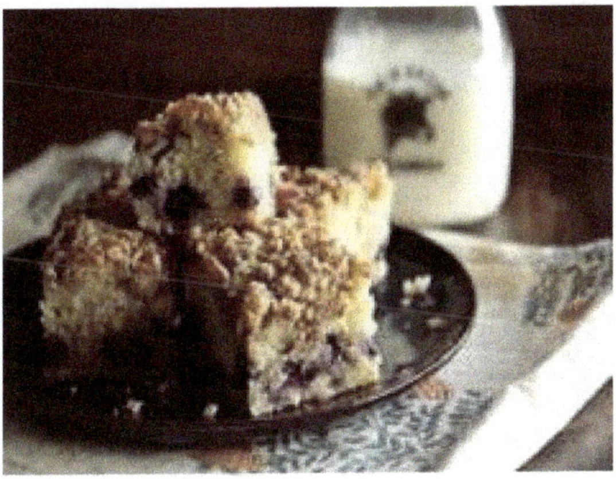

Serves: 6

Time: 40 Minutes

Calories: 381

Protein: 10 Grams

Fat: 32 Grams

Net Carbs: 20 Grams

Ingredients:

- 14 Ounces Blueberries
- 1 Tablespoon Lemon Juice, Fresh
- 1 ½ Teaspoon Stevia Powder
- 3 Tablespoons Chia Seeds
- 2 Cups Almond Flour, Blanched
- ¼ Cup Pecans, Chopped
- 5 Tablespoon coconut Oil
- 2 Tablespoon Cinnamon

Directions:

1. Mix together your blueberries, stevia, chia seeds and lemon juice, and place it in an iron skillet.
2. Mix ingredients while spreading it over your blueberries.
3. Heat your oven to 400, and then transfer it to an oven safe skillet, baking for a half hour.

Interesting Facts: Blueberries: These guys are a delectable treat that is easily incorporated into many dishes. They are packed with antioxidants and Vitamin C. Bonus: Blueberries have been proven to promote eye health and slow macular degeneration.

Rice Pudding

Serves: 6

Time: 1 Hour 35 Minutes

Calories: 330; Protein: 5 Grams; Fat: 10 Grams; Carbs: 52 Grams

Ingredients:

- 1 Cup Brown Rice
- 1 Teaspoon Vanilla Extract, Pure
- ½ Teaspoon Sea Salt, Fine
- ½ Teaspoon Cinnamon
- ¼ Teaspoon Nutmeg
- 3 Egg Substitutes
- 3 Cups Coconut Milk, Light
- 2 Cups Brown Rice, Cooked

Directions:

1. Blend all of your ingredients together before pouring them into a two quarter dish.
2. Bake at 300 for ninety minutes before serving.

Interesting Facts: Brown rice is incredibly high in antioxidants and good vitamins. It's relative, 14 white rice is far less beneficial as much of these healthy nutrients get destroyed during the process of milling. You can also opt for red and black rice or wild rice. The meal options for this healthy grain are limitless!

Pumpkin Ice Cream

(Prep time: 15 minutes/6 Servings)

Ingredients:

- 1 can coconut milk
- 1 cup unsweetened almond milk
- 1 cup canned or fresh pumpkin puree
- 1 teaspoon pure vanilla extract
- ½ teaspoon nutmeg
- 2 ½ teaspoons ground cinnamon
- ½ teaspoon ground ginger
- Pinch of salt
- 1 tablespoon gelatin

Instructions:

1. Dissolve the gelatin in ¼ cup boiling water.
2. Add the rest of the ingredients, including the gelatin mixture, to a food processor. Blend until smooth.
3. Transfer the mixture to a freezer-safe container. Cover. Freeze for 2 hours.
4. After 2 hours, use a wooden spoon to break up the ice cream in order to prevent crystalizing.
5. Leave in the freezer overnight. Serve the following day.

Nutritional Values: Carbohydrates: 4.5 grams ; Fat: 11.3 grams; Protein: 1.3 grams

Sautéed Pears

Serves: 6

Time: 35 Minutes

Calories: 220; Protein: 2 Grams; Fat: 10 Grams; Carbs: 31 Grams

Ingredients:

- 2 Tablespoons Margarine (Or Vegan Butter)
- ¼ Teaspoon Cinnamon
- ¼ Teaspoon Nutmeg
- 6 Bosc Pears, Peeled & Quartered
- 1 Tablespoon Lemon Juice
- ½ Cup Walnuts, Toasted & Chopped (Optional)

Directions:

1. Melt your vegan butter in a skillet, and then add your spices. Cook for a half a minute before adding in your pears.
2. Cook for fifteen minutes, and then stir in your lemon juice.
3. Serve with walnuts if desired.

Interesting Facts: The spice used is an absolute powerhouse and is considered one of the healthiest, beneficial spices on the plant.

Raw Vegan Chocolate Fruit Balls

Total Preparation & Cooking time: 5 mins.

Servings: 20 balls

Ingredients:

- 1/2 cup raisins
- 1 cup nuts raw cashews, almonds, macadamias
- 2 tbsp. cocoa powder, unsweetened
- 1/2 cup apricot, dried & chopped
- 1 tbsp. orange juice, fresh
- 1/2 cup organic dates, pitted & chopped
- 2 drops of natural almond essence
- 1/4 cup coconut, desiccated
- 1/2 tsp. cinnamon

Directions:

1. In a small bowl, mix the cinnamon and coconut together and keep it aside for rolling.
2. In a food processor, put all of the other ingredients, and if it doesn't get combined together completely, add in the orange juice slowly.
3. Make small balls from the mixture & coat the balls with coconut mixture.
4. Store in a refrigerator in an airtight glass container.

Nutritional Value (Amount Per Serving): 104 Calories, 5.8 g Total Fat, 0 mg Cholesterol, 12.7 g Total Carbohydrate, 2.3 g Dietary Fiber, 2.8 g Protein

CHAPTER 9: PLANT-BASED ENERGIZING DRINKS

INFUSED WATER

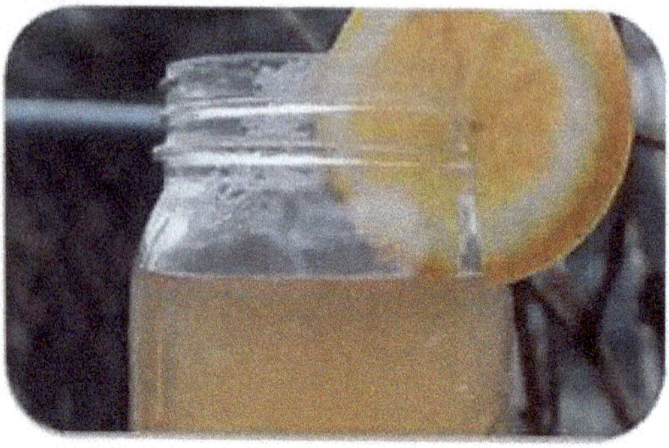

Preparation time: 5 minutes

Cooking time: 20 minutes

Total time: 25 minutes

Servings: 12

Ingredients:

- 1 lemon
- 1 orange
- 1 tbsp fresh ginger
- 5 cardamom pods
- ¼ tsp peppercorn

- 1 cinnamon stick
- 6 cups water

Directions:

1. Cut orange and lemon into slices and smash the cardamom pods. Peel the ginger and slice it up.
2. Add all ingredients to a pot and bring to a boil. Once boiling, stir and reduce the heat to a simmer. Let it simmer until the fruit slices break down.
3. Strain the liquid into a glass and serve with sugar if desired.

Nutritional Values:

- Calories 17
- Sodium 4 mg
- Total Carbs 4.3 g
- Fiber 1.3 g
- Sugar 1.6 g
- Protein 0.5 g
- Potassium 68 mg

ELIXIRS

Serves: 2

Time: 10 Minutes

Calories: 149

Protein: 3 Grams

Fat: 3 Grams

Carbs: 29 Grams

Ingredients:

- 1 Cup Riced Cauliflower, Frozen
- 1 Cup Banana, Sliced & Frozen
- ½ Cup Mixed Berries, Frozen
- 2 Cups Almond Milk, Unsweetened
- 2 Teaspoons Maple syrup, Pure & Optional

Directions:

2. Blend until mixed well.

Interesting Facts: This vegetable is an extremely high source of vitamin A, vitamin B1, B2 and B3. It has even been said that it can be used as a stress reliever!

ICED TEAS

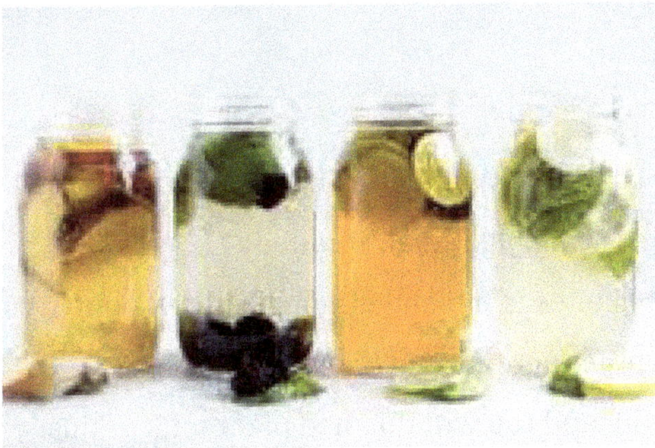

Preparation time**:** 5 minutes

Cooking time**:** 0 minutes

Total time**:** 5 minutes

Servings: 2

Ingredients:

- A cup high quality tea bag
- A tablespoon of coconut butter
- A tablespoon of plant-based milk of your choice

Optional add-ins:

- 1 teaspoon of MCT oil
- 1 teaspoon of cinnamon
- 1 teaspoon of vanilla powder

- 1 teaspoon of coconut milk powder (instead of the plant milk)

Directions:

1. Brew your coffee – either a French press or automatic coffee maker using high-quality coffee.
2. Add a cup of coffee in a blender along with coconut butter and other add-ins and blend until foamy.
3. Pour in a mug and top with foamed plant milk or dust with cinnamon.

Nutritional Values:

- Calories 73
- Total Fat 2.2 g
- Saturated Fat 0.3 g
- Cholesterol 1 mg
- Sodium 9 mg
- Total Carbs 11.7 g
- Fiber 1.6 g
- Sugar 6.2 g
- Protein2.3 g
- Potassium 235 mg

LATTE

Preparation time: 5 minutes

Cooking time: 0 minutes

Total time: 5 minutes

Servings: 2

Ingredients:

- ¼ cup almond or non-dairy milk
- 2 tbsp hemp seeds
- Splash vanilla extract
- 1.5 frozen bananas, sliced into coins
- Handful of ice
- A few pinches cinnamon
- 1 cup cooled coffee (regular or decaf)

Directions:

1. Add the ice and keep blending on high until there are no lumps remaining. Taste for sweetness and add your preferred plant-based sugar or sugar alternative.
2. Transfer to a glass and serve.

Nutritional Values:

- Calories 73
- Total Fat 2.2 g
- Saturated Fat 0.3 g
- Cholesterol 1 mg
- Sodium 9 mg
- Total Carbs 11.7 g
- Fiber 1.6 g
- Sugar 6.2 g
- Protein2.3 g
- Potassium 235 mg

CHOCOLATE

Preparation time: 5 minutes

Cooking time: 5 minutes

Total time: 10 minutes

Servings: 2 cups

Ingredients:

- 3¼ cups almond milk
- 2/3 cups semi-sweet chocolate chips
- 1½ tsp ground cinnamon
- 1/8 tsp chili powder
- 1 tsp vanilla extract
- pinch of cayenne pepper

Directions:

1. Add all ingredients to a saucepan and heat until chocolate melts.
2. Serve and enjoy.

Nutritional Values:

- Calories 931
- Total Fat 94.3 g
- Saturated Fat 82.8 g
- Cholesterol 0 mg
- Sodium 77 mg
- Total Carbs 26.4 g
- Fiber 9.7 g
- Sugar 15.3 g
- Protein 9.2 g
- Potassium 1,046 mg

MOCKTAIL

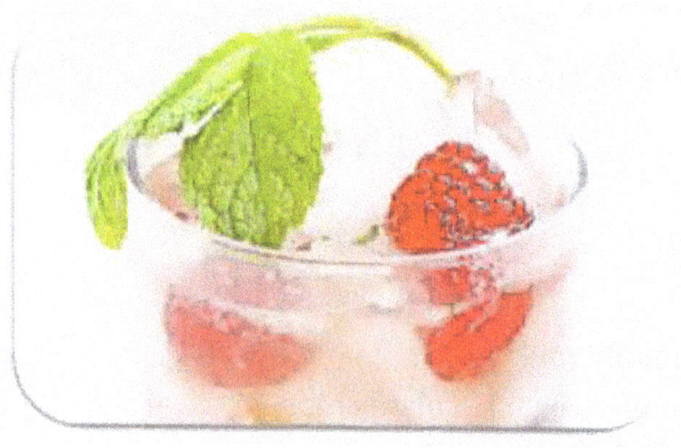

Preparation time: 15 minutes

Cooking time: 10 minutes

Total time: 25 minutes

Servings: 4

Ingredients:

- ¾ cup sugar
- ¾ cup water
- 1 package raspberries
- 1 sprig fresh mint
- 3 tbsp lime juice, freshly squeezed
- 6-8 oz sparkling mineral water
- Crushed ice

Directions:

1. To make the basic syrup, add the sugar, water, and raspberries to a saucepan over medium heat. Mix occasionally until it starts to stew. Lower the heat and delicately stew it for 5 to 7 minutes.
2. Allow cooling then strain the syrup.
3. Muddle 3 to 4 tbsp of the syrup with 1 sprig of fresh mint at the bottom of the glass.
4. Add the lime juice, sparkling mineral water, and some crushed ice to the glass and stir.

Nutritional Values:

- Calories 145
- Total Carbs 38.7 g
- Fiber 0.3 g
- Sugar 37.7 g
- Protein 0.1 g
- Potassium 27 mg

CONCLUSION

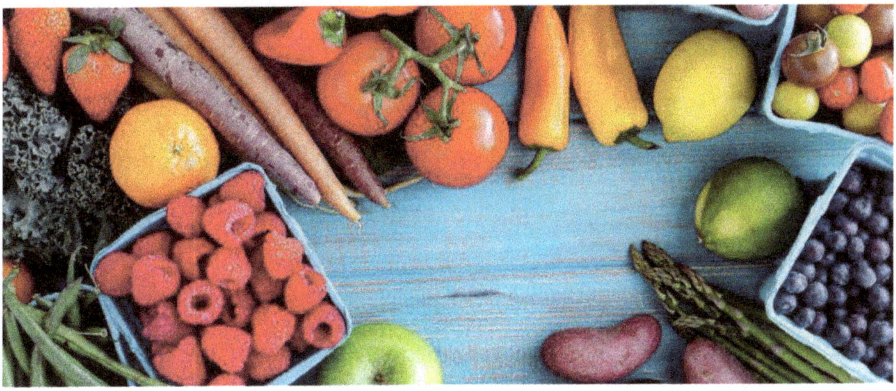

There are so many powerful and persuasive reasons to make a positive change and switch over to a plant-based diet. A plant-based diet will improve your quality of life, give you more energy and vitality, help you lose unwanted body fat, and it may even lengthen your years on this beautiful planet. As a bonus, by making the change you will be making a real and significant difference to our planet Earth's future. So much energy and fossil fuels are wasted by sourcing meat and other animal products, transporting them from place to place across miles and miles of road, and processing all of these animal products.

On top of that, there is an enormous crisis of animals being treated extremely inhumanely and cruelly. In order to mass produce meat and animal products to meet the enormous demand of the market, many manufacturers put animal comfort and quality of life last and do not make it a priority to treat them in a humane and ethical fashion.

There is also an incredible amount of food waste that happens in the production and processing of animal products. Extraordinary amounts of energy and resources are expended and too much gets simply thrown away. By switching to a plant-based diet, you will be greatly decreasing your carbon footprint and ensuring that fewer animals have to suffer at the hands of humans. And isn't that a good feeling?

Considering all the ethical reasons for switching to a plant-based diet, the enormous health benefits and improved quality of life are the icing on an already extremely appealing cake.

CPSIA information can be obtained
at www.ICGtesting.com
Printed in the USA
BVHW060037280221
601200BV00001B/28

9 781801 741170